P9-CLO-276

ALL THE
COLORS
CAME OUT

ALL THE COLORS CAME OUT

A Father, a Daughter,
and a Lifetime of Lessons

KATE FAGAN

Little, Brown and Company
New York   Boston   London

Little, Brown and Company
Hachette Book Group
1290 Avenue of the Americas, New York, NY 10104
littlebrown.com

First Edition: May 2021

Little, Brown and Company is a division of Hachette Book Group, Inc. The Little, Brown name and logo are trademarks of Hachette Book Group, Inc.

The publisher is not responsible for websites (or their content) that are not owned by the publisher.

The Hachette Speakers Bureau provides a wide range of authors for speaking events. To find out more, go to hachettespeakersbureau.com or call (866) 376-6591.

ISBN 978-0-316-70691-9
LCCN 2021930807

Printing 1, 2021

LSC-C

Printed in the United States of America

For my mom

CONTENTS

Contents

Contents

Part III

FOREWORD
by Kathy Fagan

M y grandson, Henry, with his impish grin and gorgeous blue-gray eyes, has just morphed into a heartbroken banshee. I'm not even sure what's happened. Sounds like his younger sister Frankie might have taken a bite of his granola bar. Or maybe she stole a Pokémon card out of his deck. There is no identifying what's caused this precipitous tumble to the depths of despair. A wailing, drawn-out "Nana, it's not fair" punctuates his sobs. "Oh, Henry." I lock eyes with my son-in-law, Mike. "About this fair thing. One lesson you need to learn at an early age is that life's not fair." He continues crying, ignoring this relevant and well-timed pearl of wisdom offered from grandmother to seven-year-old.

My real thought in the moment: *What's not fair, Henry, is that your grandfather isn't here to chuckle at your meltdown, tell you it's not worth crying about, and then distract you with a game of HORSE.*

That thought lives alongside others that pop up at random moments. It's not fair that Chris doesn't get to enjoy the house at

Lake George that we finally splurged on. That Chris doesn't get to be there as we celebrate Frankie's fourth birthday, and he can't rib her for changing into three different outfits just because that's what she does every day. That Chris didn't get to see Henry make those baskets during first-grade rec nights and then look over at his mom and dad with gap-toothed smile and unabashed pride. That it's me who takes him aside and tells him to always remember rule No. 1: Don't tell people how good you are. Show them.

But those are the thoughts I have when the anger surfaces, along with the cold, stark knowledge of how Chris suffered with ALS. That rage lives alongside my awe at the dignity and humor with which he endured it.

The other thoughts I have focus on fairness's first cousin (or is it a sibling?): luck. While you could say we got a heavy dose of bad luck, and that is undeniable, my heart tends toward celebrating the abundance of luck in our lives, as a couple and as a family. Chris might frown on this, because like many athletes he wasn't a big believer in luck, but he'll have to deal with it.

He loved lists, so I'll come up with one here (there will be more):

1. Luck
2. Fate
3. Kismet
4. Serendipity
5. Destiny
6. Fortune
7. Karma

Isn't it mind-boggling how much beauty and havoc these right time/right place situations, in tandem with our free will, can produce in all our lives? I'm not sure which was at play when I went to a mixer at Theta Chi my third night as a freshman at Colgate University, but it led to being asked to dance by a big, scary-looking guy with a Fu Manchu mustache and a clearly amateur bowl haircut. I guess he found my Rhode Island accent and Ann & Hope blouse alluring. I do remember that I got off the dance floor as soon as I could. We just didn't seem destined for much of anything, this big lug and me. I felt intimidated and uncomfortable, and we barely managed to make eye contact or even dance through the entirety of "Brandy (You're a Fine Girl)." A year and a half later I began to realize that we were destined. It was a sharp turn: from seeing him as a big, scary-looking stranger to appreciating the gentle but powerful forward on the basketball team. (My financial aid job was as a twelve-hour-per-week assistant to the basketball coach, and one of Chris's jobs was to help the team win.) I started always keeping an eye out for him, even while we dated other people.

I don't remember the exact moment that translated to "Do you wanna go on a date?" in January of 1976. I do remember the fun we had on that first date, the easiness of the drive from Hamilton, New York, to Auburn along Route 20 to go visit an admired assistant coach who had moved on. It was as we were approaching a major hill that he delivered a bombshell I recall to this day. "Guess what they're saying is bad for you?" "No idea, what?" "Sugar." "No way!" Yup, the life-altering moments that stick with you.

There was never a proposal in the classic sense. As a matter of fact, I was pretty much the one who proposed, in a letter written on purple stationery with pink and white flowers at the top. I must have been choosing my words carefully if I looked at the letter long enough to have the design seared into my memory. The pertinent paragraph started along the lines of "So, do you think we should get married?" It was the summer before my senior year. I was doing my summer term and he was a counselor at a camp in the Berkshires before coming back to be a graduate assistant coach for the basketball team. We were both twenty-one. In other words, the old days.

Skipping a lot of our dating experience and scooting right back to our friend luck, I offer the reasons why, at such a tender age, I thought we could make a good couple for the long haul.

1. I liked him.
2. I liked his big family. We had similar Catholic, lower-middle-class backgrounds.
3. He was an athlete (a huge factor, since my entire childhood was marinated in Boston Red Sox baseball and Providence College Friars basketball fandom).
4. He treated his mother with respect.
5. He was funny.
6. He was smart.
7. He had straight hair, so if we had girls, maybe they wouldn't struggle with curly, frizzy hair like I did (yes, this was an actual thought in my head, and we did have girls, who should thank me to this day for my foresight).

I think I loved Chris when I was twenty-one. What exactly is love at that untested, early age? Did I really know? Probably not. I know I did as we aged and struggled together. And yet, still, that's a pretty good list.

Our life as a couple was a solid one. We cruised along and hit a variety of speed bumps. Some we approached with caution so that the impact was minimal. Some we careened over at the wrong angle, and it felt like we might just fall apart. But we didn't. We never let it spiral out of control and always came back to each other and to the long view. When it was all over, didn't we want to look back on what we'd created and not what we'd let go?

And this is where luck and its variations come in again. Not from the perspective of our marriage per se, but from a more far-reaching vantage point. When we were dating and then newly married, we were so focused on us: the newness, the compatibility, the travel, the fun, the navigating of arguments. And then the diapers. Did I ever consciously factor in what kind of a father I thought he'd be? I don't think I did. My "Why I should marry him" list augured well for this, but you never really know.

Lucky us . . . our daughters hit the jackpot.

You'll read lots of stories from Kate. They're told in a far better way than I could ever muster, but here are a few snippets from my point of view.

1. Chris wasn't the biggest diaper changer and infant caregiver: "I'll do better when they can talk."
2. Ryan or Kate often rode on his shoulders until it became impossible. What you don't see from the gorgeous, stylized cover of this book is that the actual photo was taken on the rocky coast of Brittany, France, and that he carried a daughter in each arm. I know that those eyes and that smile are saying "my girls."
3. Drive time had to be filled with games he'd make up—a standard one during the holiday season had the girls taking the left or right side of the car and counting the Christmas lights on their side, the winner declared only once we'd pulled into the driveway. They would probably argue with me, but I swear this lasted into middle school. Another game that worked amazingly for a while when they were little was seeing who could keep quiet for the longest. Diabolical.
4. He sat quietly in the stands at Kate's basketball games. No yelling at the coach, no yelling at the refs, no yelling to or at her. Stoic. (I was a basket case.)

5. He was so much louder at Ryan's meets. The joy he felt at her high school and college events was palpable. He loved watching cross-country—its colorful flags and tents, crisp air, and, above all, individual grit—more than basketball.

6. Our Friday nights were always fun because he devised a way to give everyone a stake in the outcome. We gathered four pens and four pieces of paper, and each of us pondered our ideal night's entertainment. A favorite restaurant, eating at home, movie, bowling, game night, it was all up for grabs. Once we went around the horn and the itineraries were announced, they were all written down (and to the tune of a bit of lobbying). Then came the secret ballot—a simple 1 through 4 ranking. The choice with the lowest score would be the Fagan clan's evening entertainment. Sometimes this part was more fun than the evening out.

7. He suffered more from empty nest syndrome than I did.

We were allowed one last stroke of luck. Chris died on December 4, 2019, three months before the pandemic began to wreak havoc on all of us. We got the gift that none of us will ever take for granted again—the opportunity to say goodbye and hold hands and sit in companionable silence. To cry a bit more and laugh a bit more together. Friends and family came from all over to hug him and tell him what was in their hearts.

Before Kate and her wife, Kathryn, had flown back up to our area in late November for what we thought would be Chris's life-extending tracheostomy procedure, they purchased colorful bracelets for all of us and proclaimed us "Team Trach" to help Chris through the procedure and its consequences. You'll learn about how that goal fell apart. But Team Trach didn't. Once we had moved Chris through the double doors and over to the hospital room where he would die, our purpose was to make sure he felt calm and loved and had enough morphine in his system by the time we took him off life support. The doctors said that given the weakness of his lungs it would take anywhere from a few minutes to a few hours until he was gone. But then there's that indomitable human spirit, especially Chris Fagan's. We took him off life support at about 8 p.m. on Monday, December 2, still talking to him and telling our stories and holding his hands. A few hours came and went and we tired a bit and took turns sleeping in hospital chairs scattered around his bed.

When Chris was still holding on by the evening of the third we decided Mike and Ryan should head home to be with Henry and Frankie, and Kate and Kathryn needed a few hours of rest in an actual bed. I would call them as soon as anything changed.

That change came a few minutes before 1 a.m. on Wednesday morning with the first warning bell on the monitor. I texted the girls. They didn't make it in time, but I will forever be grateful for the next minutes. It was just Chris and me, this time the exact opposite of that first dance at Theta Chi. We weren't an uncomfortable five feet apart, but shared a kaleidoscopic connection, my lips to his ear. The bookends on our life together. "Hey, what an awesome time we had, didn't we?" Then the snippets that I pray somehow filled his consciousness until 1:11 a.m. and beyond. Corsica...Ryan's birth and ants on the bottle...the Breton farmhouse...Indy for Super Bowl XLVI...Cape Cod and missing the ferry to Nantucket...Fougères...the party for his fiftieth...Sweet Sixteen in Knoxville...LSU—she was an All-American!...Piana...tear gas...flyin' Baby Ryan...beating North Carolina during March Madness at Boulder...I love you...11:11...AAU trips...Giants games and soup on the stove...Dartmouth meets...we love you...thank you.

Tears are streaming down my face right now reliving this and at the same time mourning for all the families who've been denied it.

Foreword

What is it we want in the end? Is it to have been deeply loved? By many? By one? I think the ultimate gift, the proof that we were loved and profoundly, is that we're vividly remembered. Remembered the way Kate does here. Chris's drive, his devotion, and above all his attention to his daughters' dreams made our girls who they are.

I hope you enjoy Kate's love letter to her dad.

ALL THE
COLORS
CAME OUT

Prologue

RED SUEDE PUMAS

I n my closet is a pair of red suede Puma sneakers. They are low-top, the signature shoe of Walter "Clyde" Frazier, who starred for the New York Knicks in the 1960s and '70s. When I was growing up in Schenectady, New York, in the '90s, Frazier was the color commentator for the Knicks. His voice became the soundtrack of my youth, and he spoke like he played basketball: smooth, with exciting flourishes. He wore eccentric suits ("When I go to a tailor, I say, 'Show me something you think nobody would ever wear'") and peppered the broadcasts with Clydisms: *dipping and diving, juking and jiving, abounding and astounding.*

Since my family watched every game (all eighty-two in the season) for a string of years, we became accustomed to Frazier's signature flavor, most of his colloquialisms passing unremarked upon. But at least once a game, my dad would be delighted by Frazier—*swishing and dishing!*—and he'd imitate the announcer, producing as many Clydisms as he could string together without pause until they

3

became increasingly nonsensical: *praying and laying, buying and lying, sighing and frying.* I'd add in one or two; my older sister, Ryan, would smile. Then we'd keep watching the game.

My dad's appreciation for Walt Frazier was always curious to me. The two men couldn't have been more different. My dad avoided flashiness. In his mind, flashiness was desperation, which revealed insecurity. He believed, and said to me many times, that one goal in life should be for me to quietly go about my business and let people realize, on their own, how awesome I am. "Don't tell them you're great. Show them," he would say to me over and over.

Also, my dad hated suits, and he definitely never went to a tailor. His uniform was basketball shorts and a hoodie. Even at work, a family business he ran with his brother, he wore a coat and tie only on days he had meetings with clients. At six foot five, his physique drew enough attention, and he was content to duck his head and slip into the back of places.

But he loved Frazier. The guy had "put his money where his mouth is"—another thing my dad loved to say about people he admired. Walt Frazier had won an NBA title; he'd done the work. In that way, my dad's love for Frazier made sense. He respected passion; people who *went all out.* With them, he felt a kinship.

The red suede Pumas that now sit in my closet arrived at my doorstep about three years ago. I was surprised. I wasn't expecting a package, but I also knew what it was right away because sneaker boxes have a distinct shape. When I opened it and recognized the Puma logo, I thought, *Dad.* I mostly wore Nikes, and the only person (other than me) who would buy me kicks was my dad.

After I graduated from college, he started a yearly tradition: I was to select what I believed were the coolest sneakers on the market and buy a pair in his size 13. He'd give me his credit card info, and in exchange for my "fashion sense," he'd tell me to buy myself a pair, too.

Somehow, he framed this ritual as me doing him a favor, and not the other way around. He was good at that. For example, upon leaving a restaurant: "Thanks for letting me buy you dinner, Katie."

As I got older, I started to notice that sometimes he'd call upon our sneaker custom to bridge a gap between us—if he sensed I was pulling away, or too busy for him, or if he just missed me and wanted to pretend I was a kid again. I'd be trying to get off the phone, anxious to get back to my life, and he'd throw out the lifeline: "Hey, I was thinking, why don't you find us some sneakers?"

I hated, even as I let it happen, how once I started making more money and a free pair of sneakers didn't move the needle like it used to, I would forget he had asked me to find us—always *us*—a pair. A couple weeks later, he would check in about the sneakers, and I could almost hear him wondering if I would ever need him again, not just for sneakers but for anything.

The norm was me sending him a pair. But that day three years ago, he broke protocol. He'd come across a sneaker he thought was cool, one that also represented a bond we shared—*Walt "Clyde" Frazier*—so he'd bought us each a pair. I lifted the lid and parted the white wrapping paper, pulled one sneaker out of the box, held it in front of me, turned it front to side.

I hated them. *Ugh. Goddamn it.* I tucked them back into the box, called to thank my dad, and put them in my closet. About five or six months later, when I was up visiting my parents and wearing sneakers that weren't our red Pumas, my dad said, "You don't wear the ones I got us, do you?"

(Me: "What? Yes—of course. I mean—I do. I love them!")

Each time I looked in the closet for a pair of sneakers, I'd consider the red Pumas. A civil war would break out in my mind:

Me: You're going to regret not wearing them.

Also me: But I don't like them very much.

Me: Stop hurting Dad's feelings; shouldn't nostalgia and love outweigh fashion?

Also me: Yes, of course they *should*, and maybe next time they will.

When I knew my dad was going to die, and even after, those sneakers became my kryptonite. When I opened my closet, my head would explode with thoughts like little land mines, detonating across my mind. He just wanted to keep sharing things with you: *Boom*. He just wanted to feel needed by you: *Boom, boom*. How could you miss out on that moment, seeing his eyes light up when he noticed what sneakers you were wearing? *Boom, boom, boom.*

The last week of his life, I wore them every day to the hospital. But between steps, I'd look down and think that it was too little, too late. I'd made my decision, set my priorities.

I don't think my dad cared about the sneakers. But that's not how this works. The sneakers had come to symbolize our story, almost like how the icon on a desktop computer is just the representation, the interface, for the complicated program it launches.

The sneakers represented so much of what we'd built our relationship upon: him sharing his love of basketball, teaching me the game, imparting wisdom and sharing low fives, sweating and smiling together. And my failure to wear them represented the darker side of that connection: that I'd disappointed him by not loving the game as much as he did; by being gay; and that our shared stubbornness, the belief we each possessed that our ideas were always superior, had driven a wedge between us, starting when I chose a college across the country.

When I told Kathryn, she said, "Oh, I have something like that. When I was little, all I wanted was a Care Bear stuffed animal. My grandma heard that I wanted one, and so she decided to make one for me—handmade. And when she presented me with the toy, I told her that I didn't want the one she made, I wanted her to buy me one from the store."

About a year after the red Pumas arrived, when my dad was still alive, my mom and I were out for a walk and I explained my feelings about the sneakers. She said, "When you and your sister were young, my parents built you a dollhouse by hand, down to even painting the small figurines inside the rooms. I know they wanted to connect with you girls because we had moved away, and they felt they weren't seeing you as much, and they wanted to do something special. They were so excited to give it to us, but they didn't know you and your sister were interested in other things, and so that dollhouse was almost never played with."

These stories didn't make the red Pumas any less radioactive. They just made me realize that most people have their pair of sneakers, or handmade Care Bear, or dollhouse—an item that has come to represent, for them, a complicated relationship dynamic.

I still see these sneakers every day, on the second shelf of my closet. And every morning my chest tightens, and I usually reach out and touch the soft suede along the heel. But I never wear them. The thought of wearing them haunts me. It's not that I want to keep them pristine; it's that I don't want them reminding me, all day long, of the ways in which I failed at living up to the promise of our relationship.

PART

I

Chapter 1

US

I was the daughter of an athlete. I knew that from the beginning.

Every so often when I was a kid, if a guy didn't know us very well, he might ask my dad if he wished he had sons. My dad would look at the guy with bewilderment. "Not ever, not once," he'd say, then look at me and wink. Usually, he'd lean over and whisper to me, "You should hear the answer I give when you're not here," grinning while offering a conciliatory, and conspiratorial, low five before I could even scowl.

This was the first lesson he ever taught me: Value your teammates. And my dad and I, we were on the same team. I knew this from the beginning, too, and I knew it especially—given everything we went through along the way—at the very end.

Christopher John Fagan—aka Dad, aka Daddio, aka The Big C—always considered himself an underdog, and he would tell me stories about how he fought his way onto the varsity basketball team at his Catholic high school, then into the starting lineup at Colgate

University, and finally onto professional teams across Europe. He was the oldest of six kids—three boys and three girls—who grew up in a small house in Troy, New York, about three hours up the Hudson River from Manhattan. The house had one room for the boys, one for the girls, and visiting my dad's "cozy" childhood home helped me understand why he seemed addicted to always having someone around.

On the court, he made his dreams happen despite almost dying of kidney failure the summer before his sophomore year of high school, the doctors telling his parents he wouldn't survive the night, a priest standing over his bed and delivering last rites. Sometimes I'd forget this story, because he had no lasting health issues, but he wore the dialysis scars like a badge of honor, and later I'd occasionally appreciate that he probably believed he could duplicate this result—once again snatch life from the jaws of death.

When I was just a kid, my dad would show me the route he would run in his blue-collar neighborhood, from his childhood home and back. I loved these pilgrimages; like visiting Penny Lane or Strawberry Fields or something. *This is where greatness was forged.* We'd be in his car, windows down, rolling toward a stop sign, and I could picture my dad, lithe and young, in his floppy Converses. This was the beginning of my education about what dreams actually are. They're hard work. They're a shimmering blacktop in the summer heat. I'd stare out at the pavement and wonder if I had what it took, or if maybe there were other dreams that weren't so daunting to achieve.

Each morning, when he lifted his large body out of bed, he would say aloud, "Power, strength, and mental toughness." According to this belief system, nothing existed that couldn't be overcome through willpower and perseverance. I know his morning mantra because my mom heard him say it thousands of times. The two of them met at Colgate, at a frat party. She and her two sisters grew up outside Providence, Rhode Island, in a single-story home on the flight path to T. F. Green Airport. My mom and dad had many things in common, including a love of sports and parents who appreciated the value of a dollar, which shaped their shared belief that they were salt-of-the-earth.

At Colgate, my dad was on the basketball team, and this was the 1970s, so his brown hair sat atop his head like an upside-down bowl, and a Fu Manchu mustache hung from his face. My mom thought he looked like a picture she'd once seen in a history book, a picture of Genghis Khan.

But that comparison isn't quite right, because my dad was tall, with long legs, and no propensity toward violence—though when you turned his dial just right, his anger could wilt you. She was a foot shorter than he, and their wedding pictures are adorable, with my dad seeming to hunch ever so slightly in each one of them. Or maybe it's a trick of the eye, because I spent so many years watching him tilt his head to come down the stairs.

My sister, Ryan, was born in 1980 on the island of Corsica, where my dad was playing for a team in Ajaccio. I was born a year later, in Rhode Island, a factoid I could never get over. How did they manage to birth my sister on an exotic island south of France, earning her dual citizenship, while having me in...Rhode Island?

After having spent five seasons abroad, my dad playing for various teams across Europe, my parents settled, two kids in tow, outside of Albany, New York, where the sprawling Fagan family all still lived. Though he rarely dressed the part, my dad's work was actually white collar: he was a financial advisor alongside his brother, Dennis, at their family investment firm, Fagan Associates. My dad mostly made his own hours, which was helpful because my mom worked as a textbook sales representative for McGraw-Hill, traveling to colleges and universities and frequently spending nights on the road.

Our childhood was awesome. My sister and I had no complaints. Looking back, my parents struck a lovely balance between authoritarianism and democracy. I never thought my parents were my friends, per se, but I really liked them and was happy to run up and give them a hug, even at school functions where high schoolers seemed to believe adults were an embarrassment.

Ryan eventually ran cross-country at Dartmouth. Beginning in seventh grade, Dad would attend her races looking like he could be a coach, wearing the school sweatshirt and a Timex watch, but he was nothing of the kind. And he liked that he knew little of Ryan's sport; he had no preconceived notions about how she should be doing things.

When it came to basketball, he knew it all. I actually don't even remember him teaching me how to shoot—it must have been in first grade—but as I got older, I reaped the benefits of his mastery. Learning a skill that young created the illusion of inheritance, as if I didn't learn to play so much as the knowledge already existed inside me. I excelled in high school, accepted a scholarship to play at the University of Colorado, and played three years professionally. Basketball, and sports, became the beating heart of my life.

And it took me everywhere. Until I was thirty-five years old, I didn't live in the same apartment for longer than a year. A sampling of the places I lived: Colorado, Ireland, Washington State, Philadelphia, New York, and, finally, with Kathryn, Charleston, South Carolina. After basketball, I crisscrossed the country working for newspapers, eventually landing a job at the *Philadelphia Inquirer* covering the 76ers of the NBA, which springboarded me to ESPN.

Over the years, Ryan lived in New York and Boston—always within striking distance of family. Eventually she and her husband, Mike, settled in a town outside of Boston and had two kids: Henry, then Francesca. My mom and dad visited them every other weekend until, in 2018, Ryan moved her family back to our hometown to be near our parents.

My dad was always terrified of dying, perhaps because he'd once come so close. He would not speak of death, even on the occasion of someone else's. And when a body appeared on our TV screen— the kind thoughtfully tended to, or just in a casket—he would stand up from the couch and excuse himself to go to my parents' upstairs bedroom, and we would be left to decide: turn off the show, put on a ball game, or continue even in the face of his protest?

Even as a kid I recognized his fear, and for many years it made him mortal. Otherwise, he was like my personal superhero: He could toss me onto his shoulders or launch me into a pool; he was really witty and smart, and he was the best basketball player I'd ever seen. I was the sidekick he draped an arm across and sent on special missions, like into the convenience store to get us Gatorade.

As I got older, in my late twenties, and began seeing my parents more clearly, as most kids eventually do, I realized my dad's fear of death was actually fear of separation. He could not imagine being gone from us, or us from him. His religion had been movement, sweat a daily offering. This, along with his ruthless practicality—*I'll believe it when I see it*—kept him away from organized faith, including the Catholicism of his youth. As far as he could tell, death was final, and he saw no reason to think about something so awful.

Chapter 2

BROKEN ARM(S)

My mom was actually the one with big dreams. She was the one who, growing up, fell asleep at night picturing a life that touched down in foreign countries, that cut across cultures. When she was young, she read *Nicholas and Alexandra*, about the Romanovs, the last royal family of Imperial Russia, and she became obsessed with the country—its terrible juxtaposition of opulence and cruelty. From then on, she dreamt of becoming NBC's foreign correspondent in Russia. She pictured standing outside the Kremlin in a knit hat and down coat and beaming home news about Russia's latest mischief on the world stage.

In fact, one summer while at Colgate University, my mom worked at the local TV news station in Utica, New York. She once told me about an assignment she'd received, covering the opening of a runaway truck ramp. She told me about how she'd stood at the base of the steep gravel incline and pointed upward, explaining to her viewers how a truck with failed brakes could pull off the paved road and find blessed relief, and safety, in the extreme gradient.

I remember this story because I laughed and laughed. I said, "Okay, so, you—my *mom*—covered the grand opening of…a runaway truck ramp?" She could not recall, despite my prodding, the exact words she used to convey this information to the local audience. But seared into my memory is the image of my mom, microphone in hand, at the base of the slope, injecting her voice with gravitas. Ever since, when I pass a runaway truck ramp—a frequent occurrence on the winding roads of the Northeast—I think of my mom and her broadcasting dreams, which never quite made it up their own steep hill.

My dad, as far as I gleaned, never had desires like these coursing through his veins. He was provincial. He dreamed of a good game of basketball, a crisp fall day with a football game, a couple of kids he could take with him everywhere. Even playing basketball overseas, even this was fueled by my mom's wanderlust, her hunger for adventure. My dad never needed travel and high-cost hopes, but he was thrilled that his twenty-two-year-old bride was encouraging him to play hoops for a third of the money he could have made at home.

If they hadn't met at Colgate, if they hadn't started a family, perhaps my mom might have tried to become a national TV reporter. But when she and my dad left for Europe, she felt that very little could be done in pursuit of her own dreams, and by the time they returned they had not one, but two children.

Images of those years in France flicker across my mind like scenery out a train window: the white Tom & Jerry shirt I loved and wore everywhere; an afternoon at Mont St. Michel; a bag of fresh chocolate croissants; an afternoon watching *The Mask of Zorro* and making crepes; sitting in the bleachers, my dad on the court in his blue shorts and unruly mustache; my sister singing in French at a school assembly; the cartoon *Bibifok* (pronounced "Baby Fuck"), about a baby seal, the theme song of which Ryan and I would go around singing—"Bibi, bibi, bibi…foc"—causing my mom and dad to grimace at each other.

One year, around 1985, when my sister was five years old, so I was four, my dad was playing in Fougères, in Brittany. That winter he was recovering from a broken right arm. My dad never had much compassion for referees, especially not the ones in France, who seemed to have a cultural vendetta against American players— at least, so felt my dad. After one particularly testy game, during which my mom watched her husband constantly complaining to the referees, she advised him to chill out. He wasn't doing himself any good. And worse, he was getting a bad rap. And so, the next game, instead of yelling at the ref, my dad took out his irritation on the padded pole beneath the basket. The padding, though, was more aesthetic than functional, and his arm fractured with the impact.

Because of this chain of events, my mom felt personally invested in his rehabilitation, which included going to the gym with him at all hours and rebounding so he could more quickly return to game shape. It was just the four of us, so Ryan and I would tag along and entertain ourselves, which wasn't hard. An empty gymnasium with rows of bleachers? The space was a blank canvas for our imaginations.

I wish I could remember the day it happened—the day Ryan fell off the side of the bleachers. The gym in Fougères was ancient. The bleachers were concrete, no railings. In fact, everything was rock solid except the wooden basketball floor. Ryan and I were playing on the row above the team locker rooms, which were down a flight of stairs into the basement. It was into this opening that my sister fell, technically two flights, onto the jagged landing of the steps.

My mom and dad were on the court, their focus elsewhere. I guess I yelled, and they came racing over. Ryan had a broken arm, which in retrospect was incredibly lucky. (Worth noting: My dad's displeasure with referees cost our family two broken arms. And, no, he didn't learn his lesson.) I have heard this story dozens of times. And I'm just now recognizing, literally as I write this, that it was always my mom doing the telling—her voice suggesting guilt—as if the burden of caretaking was hers, not his; the injury her failure of parenting, not theirs. My dad would always add a little spice to the story, a quip here and there, but I got the sense that in his memory he believed he was precisely where he was supposed to be—on the court.

It's curious, how guilty my mom feels about this long-ago broken arm. Sometimes I can't decipher if she's truly ashamed or playing at it—kowtowing to how society expects a woman to react when an untended child is injured. My mom understands that most modern parents cannot fathom leaving two young kids unsupervised in the bleachers. Whenever the story was told, my focus was on the court, picturing my mom chasing down rebounds for her best friend. I saw my parents in a partnership, one helping the other do what he adored. Why would I want it any other way? We had parents who held us steady without holding us still.

Ryan was older, by exactly fourteen months, but we never had that traditional older-younger sibling dynamic. We always seemed to complement each other's deficiencies. She was rail thin; I was chubby. She had eyeglasses as thick as bottles; I had 20/20 vision. I had better hand-eye coordination and was more naturally athletic, but she possessed more willpower and endurance. We just seemed to work together.

Also, my sister was impossible to fight with. All you need to know about our relationship can be summed up in one detail: as kids, she offered me lifetime shotgun. The rule of shotgun, as I learned it, was that whoever first called "Shotgun!" upon stepping outside earned the coveted place in the front seat. So, once we were old enough, if we were going somewhere with just one parent, I'd race outside ahead of Ryan and scream *"Shotgun!"*—then dart around to the front seat. A few seconds later, Ryan would patiently walk out the door and climb into the back. One day, when I was buckling in, she said, "Kate, you don't need to scream 'Shotgun' every time we get into the car. You can just...have shotgun."

My head whipped around. "Are you saying I can have *lifetime* shotgun?"

"Yes," she said, unbothered, a book on her lap.

"You mean to say that, for the rest of our lives, I can always sit in the front seat?"

"Yes," she said. "Sitting in the front seat is not something I care about."

She was probably ten years old at the time.

I told this story at her wedding, and everyone recognized it as quintessential Ryan. She has never been interested in bickering, or conflict, and she perpetually offers everyone the benefit of the doubt. I've never met someone less judgmental, which makes gossiping with her hopeless.

Her constitution is one reason for our peaceful relationship. Another is that we never needed to fight for our parents' attention. Ryan started running cross-country in seventh grade, and she quickly became really good. After all, her superpowers were endurance, willpower, and intellect. Within months my dad became obsessed with the sport, to the extent that if Ryan wanted to run at night, he'd sometimes drive alongside her with the high beams on, lighting the way.

One morning the three of us were together in the car before a really important cross-country race. Ryan and my dad were strategizing: Should she go to the front of the pack early? Or should she conserve energy and try making up ground during the middle of the race? I think I was feeling left out, and mischievous, so I said something like, "Why don't you just run to the front and stay there? That seems like the best strategy."

In response, my dad looked at me in the rearview mirror to gauge my sincerity. (I think I was serious; I didn't know much about running.) Ryan shot me a look but then let it go. She was too smart to let my stupidity affect her.

My dad talked about winning insofar as we wanted to talk about winning. If Ryan expressed belief that she could finish first, and wanted his help, then he engaged. But he never encouraged us to prioritize being the winner. We were naturally competitive with each other— what family isn't?—but winning wasn't my dad's driving principle.

While working at ESPN, I'd read the same trope over and over: about how some superstar athlete "couldn't stand losing" and that he "needed to win, even at Monopoly." I never felt this kind of anecdote explained anything about the athlete's psyche. Only the least competitive among us remain docile when given the chance to beat our parents (or siblings) in a family board game. I could walk off the court after a game, and if I'd tried hard or played well, or both, I usually felt fine. The only time this wasn't true was when I played one-on-one against my dad; when he beat me, I often lost my mind.

The only edict my dad delivered when it came to sports was that we try hard, that we care. That was his line in the sand. Of this, Ryan never needed reminding. She seemed preprogrammed to get every drop out of her natural abilities—although even that phrasing isn't giving her enough credit. My sister just worked really hard, all the time, whether she was being watched or not. I was more likely to dive onto the floor if I noticed someone watching, then lollygag when they turned away. My dad recognized this tendency when I was young, around twelve years old, and he called me out on it. I promised myself it would never happen again, and it didn't. (But whenever I dove onto the floor, I would think about how everyone watching must think I'm so scrappy, which always made me feel slightly disingenuous.)

The week my parents brought me to college in Colorado, my dad and I worked out together at the campus rec center. On the last day, we played one-on-one. This would be the final time we played together before I started college basketball. He didn't do it often, but if my dad wanted to beat me—he was six five, after all—he would back me down until he was under the rim and I was powerless to stop him. Our unspoken agreement, ever since I'd been little, was that he would mostly shoot from the outside. But over the years, on the final point of a game he really wanted to win, he'd use his size.

I wasn't particularly hotheaded otherwise, but when my dad beat me, sometimes I felt such heightened emotions—a cocktail of anger, annoyance, disappointment, exasperation—that I'd pick up the basketball and throw it as hard as I could against the wall. I remember it felt good. And on these occasions, my dad would look at me with something akin to pride. That day at Colorado, my dad beat me, and those same feelings exploded in my chest. I walked off the court and spotted his stuff, which included a pair of black Oakley sunglasses. I took two more steps, then planted my left foot and soccer-kicked his sunglasses across the gym, where they exploded against the far wall.

I froze. I'd just destroyed two hundred dollars' worth of merchandise. I walked along the baseline and collected the various pieces. One lens had gone into the neighboring court, and I excused myself to those playing on it, darting into the lane to retrieve the curved, tinted piece of plastic. Then I jogged to my dad with the plastic remains in my upturned palm like a dismembered G.I. Joe. I sunk down next to him, our backs against the gym's padded wall.

"I'm sorry," I said, gently trying to reinsert the lens into the frame.
"It's okay," he said. "Don't worry about it."

"But I think maybe I can fix them," I said. I examined the dis-
lodged arm: the tiny screw, the one that would reconnect the arm to
the frame, was missing. I scanned the courts, but the screw was the
size of a Tic Tac, the gym the size of an airplane hangar.

"Seriously, don't worry about it," he said with a smile. "It's worth it
just to know this"—he gestured between us—"still matters to you."

Chapter 3

GIRL DAD

I wasn't the coolest little kid. I kept my hair cut short to be like my Little League teammates, who were all boys. During elementary school, I can remember once going to dinner at the Ground Round with my dad and the hostess saying to him, "Where would you and your son like to sit?" I dropped my eyes as my dad corrected the woman. Then, perhaps to make me feel better about this social catastrophe, he bought me the sundae they served in a plastic baseball helmet.

I was embarrassed by myself, but somehow my dad never seemed to be. He took me everywhere. From as early as I can remember, he would bring me to his nightly pickup basketball game. At first, I vaguely remember having a coloring book and wedging myself into the bleachers. A few years later, I would wait patiently for the end of each game, then dart onto the court and get some shots in while the guys went to the water fountain. I can still picture my dad, dripping sweat, helping me get in a couple shots between games.

By the time I was eleven or twelve, I was allowed to play if only nine guys showed up. Picture me sitting on the bleachers, feigning ambivalence but secretly praying for my magic number—they'd have no choice but to let me in the game. (Better the kid than no game at all!) Finally, and I'm not sure what the trigger was, my dad walked into the gym and announced that I would be playing from then on, regardless of how many guys showed up. The guy who ran the game balked, saying, "But she hasn't paid," and in response my dad grabbed his wallet, which he had tucked into his basketball sneakers, and pulled out a twenty-dollar bill. The guy pocketed the bill, defeated. A minute later, as we sat side by side tying our sneakers, I said, "Wow, Dad, thank you," and he winked and said, "You're already better than half these guys, anyway."

He never believed he deserved a badge of honor for treating me fairly. His logic was simple. He took pleasure in sharing with me the things he loved, and sports were atop the list. Much later, I realized that versions of this father-daughter interaction were being repeated across the country, as millions of young girls came of age in the 1990s, when playing sports wasn't just begrudgingly accepted but actually…cool.

Perhaps there was a time, when I was really young, when he had to encourage me to join. But I don't remember it. As far as I remember, everything went unsaid. The sound of his dresser drawer opening meant he was putting on basketball shorts; the way he dropped onto the couch and tugged on his socks meant we were leaving soon; the sound of the keys jingling as he slipped the lanyard over his neck meant it was go-time. Back then, I had no historical perspective. I did not think of myself as part of a cultural revolution or the illustration of a modern father-daughter relationship. I knew only that every night my dad grabbed his sneakers and walked out to the car and that he expected me to find the ball in the front hall closet and hop in beside him. I knew nothing if I didn't know this.

Within my childhood, different eras existed. When I was really young, I was the sidekick who tagged along while my dad played. Then came the in-between era, when I wasn't a kid but couldn't yet hold my own. My favorite era began when I was thirteen years old, when my dad realized we were a self-sustaining unit. We didn't need a pickup game. We could go to the gym, play one-on-one, shoot, run drills, and both of us could have fun.

It was during this era that my dad started sprinkling in his life philosophies without me knowing. He would smuggle these ideas into the middle of a game or a shooting drill. Some sank in right away, while the full wisdom of others unfurled over years.

Lesson #1

NEVER LET ANYONE WIN

I lost to my dad hundreds of times before I won. It's for that reason that I can still remember the exact play I made to beat him for the first time. We were playing in our driveway, and I was eleven years old. He was having a bad shooting day, which gave me a fighting chance, because I could dart all around the court getting rebounds at which he, lumbering along with his big frame, had no chance.

My game-winning basket: I drove around him to the right and did a fancy—for me, at that age—reverse lay-up that I'd been practicing for weeks. Game over. The ball dropped through the hoop and rolled to a stop in the grass. It was a summer day, I'm sure, because we'd taken a quick break from mowing the lawn to play the game.

"I won," I said, baffled, wondering what it meant. Was I an adult now? I took a long, deep breath, surprised the air still tasted the same.

"You won," he said. "Fair and square. Promise me something, though, okay? Promise me that you'll return the favor. When I get old,

I don't want you letting me win—at anything. Not because you feel sorry for me or you think you need to take pity on me, or for any reason at all. Deal?"

That sounded preposterous—these future versions of us that I couldn't conjure. Like the plot of a sci-fi movie. And yet, I could promise him; I could live by the code he was proposing.

"Why?" I asked.

"Why what?"

"Why don't you ever let me win?"

"Do you want me to let you win?"

"Well—no," I said.

"Why?" he asked back.

"Why what?"

"Why don't you want me to let you win?"

"Because that would be a lie. You'd be lying to me."

He nodded, then looked at the ball, idle in the grass, next to the pole—a still life.

"Rematch?" he said.

Chapter 4

MALIBU GRILL

My dad and I realized that my basketball dreams came true on the same day, and probably at the same moment. It was the summer before my senior year in high school, and we were at the 1998 AAU Nationals in Indianapolis, the final showcase event before colleges decided who they wanted to recruit. A series of images from that trip: a tornado warning cutting short a game during which I couldn't seem to miss, a fax from Duke University waiting for me at the front desk of our hotel, a voice mail on our room's phone from a coach at the University of Colorado, my dad inside a gas station pay phone calling home with the good news, and a lunch between games at a restaurant called Malibu Grill.

We sat across from each other at a freestanding table in the middle of the restaurant and my dad said, "It's happening; you made it happen—wow, a college scholarship." He was never overly animated, so I just remember him stirring sugar into his iced tea, smiling slyly at me, and my distinctly feeling that there was no daylight between my exhilaration and his. He paid for the meal and slipped the receipt into his tattered black wallet. During my senior year of high school, that lunch at Malibu Grill was folklore between us, the mere suggestion of it conjuring feelings of conquering heroes: the day father and daughter broke bread with the basketball gods. It was our historic landmark; I pictured a plaque outside: *On these premises, in July of 1998…*

By my senior year of college, very little was the same. I'd been gone—1,800 miles away—for five years, but the actual physical distance seemed shorter than the emotional gulf. I'd come out as gay (to my mom), but still couldn't manage a face-to-face conversation about it with my dad.

Yet at the end of my senior season at Colorado, my parents and grandparents flew out for my final home game, where the school honors families at center court and the seniors get to say a little something to the crowd after the game. That night we all ended up at the Cheesecake Factory in downtown Boulder, the six of us at a table in the back of the restaurant, the place mostly cleared out. My dad was sitting across from me. When the bill came, he took out his wallet and placed a credit card on the tab, then looked at me and slid a worn sliver of paper across the table.

"What is it?" I said, tentatively reaching for it.

"Take a look." He leaned back.

I touched the paper, its corners frayed. I unfolded it and started from the bottom. First, I saw my dad's signature, a scribble I'd recognize anywhere. Then my eyes scanned upward, and I saw the total: $17.93. Above that was the itemized list of purchases: club sandwich, Caesar salad, iced tea, and Diet Coke. And then, above that, I saw the words I'd secretly been hoping to see. At the top of the receipt, centered, in print that had already started to fade, it read MALIBU GRILL.

I looked at my dad. His eyes were soft. He shrugged instead of saying anything because nothing said more than the paper in my hand. And that night at the Cheesecake Factory, I was reminded that he wanted my dreams for me as much as I wanted them for myself.

Chapter 5

MARCH MADNESS

In my family we observed the traditional holidays, but when I was around twelve years old, my dad added one: March Madness. Days off school are always nice, but the fact I had two that were just mine felt sacred, and I remember waking up on those mornings and sensing the shimmering dawn of my independence.

It all began on a Wednesday, the night before the opening game of the NCAA tournament, round about 1992. I was playing pickup with my dad, and we started talking about the brackets, the best matchups, and I realized the games I most wanted to watch were played during the school day. Very few sporting events took place during working hours, usually just global events like the Olympics and the World Cup, and I remember believing the schedule of the NCAA tournament was cruel and unfortunate.

We were sitting on the low row of bleachers when my dad seemed to alight on a solution to a problem that, just seconds before, seemed impenetrable.

"Oh," he said. "You just won't go."

"What?"

"Yeah, that sounds like a good plan, doesn't it?"

"I can just...skip school?"

"Well, it's not really skipping school, is it? We have a reason, and a very good reason, and I don't see why school should keep you from learning—even if it's a different kind of learning. That would be backward and against the idea of education, right?" This was the same man I once saw sitting on the edge of his bed, his face contorted in pain as he tried to wriggle his severely sprained ankle into a dress shoe so he wouldn't miss a day of work. We weren't a family in the business of playing hooky—or so I thought.

"Ultimately, the school doesn't know what's best for you, we do," he said. "And all I hoped for you and Ryan is that you'd find something you love and work hard at it. And you're doing that. I'm not sure what a perfect record at school proves to anyone except that you know how to follow rules—and that'll only get you so far. So, yeah, I think no school tomorrow, or Friday, and we watch the games together."

When I think of my March Madness holidays, my next thought is always the song "No Surrender" by Bruce Springsteen: "We learned more from a three-minute record, baby, than we ever learned in school." In my case, I learned more while missing class—about responsibility and freedom and how they're intertwined—than I ever did in school.

And from that Wednesday night in 1992 until the year I went to college, I would stay home on the first two days of the NCAA tournament and watch the games with my dad. The beginning of this tradition also marked the establishment of a new household policy: I was allowed to take mental health days or go in to school an hour late anytime I deemed necessary.

Included in this rule, but never explicitly stated, was that I never abuse the privilege. It's strange, how seriously I took this. Before, I'd mischievously hold a thermometer to a lightbulb, trying to stage a fever, or just complain for no reason about being tired. But suddenly I was empowered. My choices were mine. And given this authority, I realized I had to ask myself what kind of person I wanted to be. Not all off-days were created equal: some were earned and felt peaceful; others were stolen and stoked guilt.

There were about twelve years between the end of my college career and his ALS diagnosis, yet I can only remember watching the tournament together once. Not for lack of trying on his part. He invited me to join him in Vegas, he offered to drive down to New York, he asked if I wanted to come up. Not a year passed without him trying to re-create the father-daughter magic of March Madness, est. 1992.

I knew what he was doing. And I knew what I was doing—that is, testing fate—each time I presented my *very busy life* as an excuse for why I couldn't get together with him. There are other interactions I regret, but mostly because I'm projecting my adult perspective onto them, wishing I could go back and say or do something revealed to me only over time. So those moments aren't regret as much as disappointment—a burning, a knowing. March Madness leaves me scorched with shame. I knew I was throwing away something special. I could hear that voice, my own, pressing on my heart, urging me to listen. And I silenced it with lame excuses. (*Work, busy, no time, next year, love you.*)

I don't even fill out a bracket anymore. When I was on *Around the Horn*, a TV show on ESPN, I had to join their pool, and I picked the games with my eyes closed. Those brackets took me less than two minutes, though when I was growing up, my dad and I would pore over them for hours, and I took great pride in having a legitimate explanation for each of my selections.

My dad decided to break the rules of achievement culture so we could spend time together. When I got older, I handed that power right back.

Chapter 6

TOO MUCH ALIKE

In July of 2016, I walked into my dad's hospital room with Kathryn, who at the time was my girlfriend, a few minutes after he'd woken up from surgery. He was sitting up, smiling, his pale yellow gown twisted and barely covering everything that needed to be covered. But he wasn't concerned. His energy was upbeat, which I quickly understood was caused by the drugs. My mom was in a chair next to him.

At fifty-nine years old, my dad had already played two lifetimes of basketball. The disks in his neck were pressing together, pinching the nerves, which in turn was affecting his left hand—or so the doctor believed. It was the kind of diagnosis my dad, a practical man, understood: behavior X causes Y and is alleviated by Z. He'd long ago accepted that playing hoops through middle age would take its toll, and he considered this neck operation—along with his previous hip replacement and rotator cuff surgery—the price of admission.

We all welcomed the surgery. Chalk this up to the theory of

relativity, considering the other explanation floated for my dad's symptoms: ALS. We would learn only later that many ALS patients are first diagnosed with neck compression. (It seems even doctors are desperate to avoid delivering this brutal diagnosis.)

"Ka-tie!" he said, loopy, his voice still raspy from being under.

"Hi, Dad," I said, squinting, putting on that jokey, tentative voice you use when someone you love is acting strangely. (*What's gotten into you!*) His eyes moved past me to the door, and I turned to see a nurse walking to his bedside. I was not surprised to learn they'd already developed a rapport but shocked when he said to her, "This is my daughter Kate and her girlfriend, Kathryn," since I don't think he'd ever before introduced someone as my girlfriend. I knew he really liked Kathryn. I resisted the urge to go wrap him in a bear hug.

Kathryn had appeared in my life overnight, though it took me a few months to take her intentions seriously. We met in Southern California, at the annual espnW Women and Sports Summit, at a fancy hotel on the ocean. We were both there for work: I to moderate panels; she to teach yoga each morning to attendees. I took Kathryn's crowded outdoor class; the air from the ocean was salty, and her beauty was like a yoga advertisement brought to life. She was charismatic and kind, and I assumed she was also straight. She "seemed" straight, anyway—I had almost no experience with sexuality as fluid. In women's sports, too often, you needed an answer: gay or not gay? Not many women moved freely between the two worlds.

We exchanged a few words after her class, and then after the night-time cocktail party, one of her friends pulled me aside and seemed to imply that Kathryn had a crush on me. I kept one eye on Kathryn for the rest of the night but had this underlying, irrational worry that a prank was being pulled. I reasoned she was too beautiful to like me. That night we talked for a few minutes and danced near, but not with, each other, and the next morning we exchanged cell numbers before she left to teach in San Francisco.

She texted me from her Uber on the way to the airport, and I don't think we've stopped texting since. She was unexpected in almost every way: her forthrightness about her feelings, her stereo-typically feminine appearance that belied an inner tomboy who'd grown up stalking Cobi Jones of Team USA soccer and point guard Jacque Vaughn of the University of Kansas, and her salt-of-the-earth sensibility, which she wraps in poufy haute couture.

Until I met Kathryn, I'd been in a string of relationships that were never quite what I wanted. Along the way, I started to believe I couldn't have everything. As a gay woman, my pool of potential partners was limited. It was a numbers game, plain and simple. If you believe that about 4 percent of Americans are lesbian, gay, or bisexual, then cut that in half for gender—well, you start to see how perhaps the options are narrower.

In the year before we met, I had this theory that relationships are like gymnastics routines. Not all have the same starting value. Some routines are designed to be safe, so that the gymnast can feel secure and execute what they know they're capable of. These routines have a starting value of 7 out of 10, perhaps 8—meaning that even if the gymnast executes everything perfectly, the highest score possible is still mediocre. I'd been in relationships where even if everything went as well as possible—and how often does everything go "as well as possible"?—we could manage a barely passing grade. Our starting value just wouldn't allow anything higher.

From the moment I met Kathryn, I knew she was the daring, risky routine. That for the two of us, together, our starting value was 10. Smart, kind, charming, funny, beautiful, and self-sufficient, she was the kind of partner I'd dreamed of. And that was scary, because that meant she was also the kind of partner who, if I ever lost her, would hollow out my insides. She could break my heart. Wouldn't it be better to pull things back and just go for the safety of a 7?

People know. They know, deep down, even as they're standing up there at the altar in front of everyone, when they've lowered the starting value—dropped the triple backflip from their routine. And they can feel it every day of the relationship. What I feel with Kathryn, perhaps more than anything else, is lucky. I am lucky to be given the chance at such a marriage.

At first blush, my dad and Kathryn had little in common. She is short, five foot two, loves fantasy novels and mysticism, and spent the first half of her career teaching yoga around the world. Meanwhile, Dad couldn't touch his toes, and skeptical was his default setting. But what they both had, among other things, was a curiosity about other people and an abiding appreciation of nature. My dad was instantly smitten with the duality that is Kathryn. He connected with her midwestern sensibility—she had grown up in Lawrence, Kansas— and that foundation allowed him to willingly explore other aspects of her, like yoga, and crystals, and the universe's lucky numbers.

They first met in early 2016, in New York City. Even when healthy, my dad was hobbled. He didn't walk so much as lumber. And on this day, as we strolled the streets of Manhattan, my dad fell behind, as he often did. I was walking with my mom, and we were chatting. At a streetlight, I paused and turned around and saw, a block behind us, Kathryn and my dad, the two of them laughing and talking. His appreciation of her was instantaneous and adorable, and the first time we went upstate to visit them, my dad proudly had on display a few copies of her book, *Aim True,* which he would show to anyone who stopped by the house.

On the day of his neck surgery, the nurse left after a few pleasantries and I looked back at my dad, who was oblivious to the fact that he'd done something noteworthy in introducing Kathryn as my girlfriend. He looked me in the eye and, his tone as openly curious as if he'd been meaning to ask me all my life, said, "Do you think we're just too much alike? Is that what's always bogged us down?"

Everything screeched to a halt. Picture me like a character in a show who learns some fact that upends their worldview and everything goes into superspeed rewind—oceans sailed in reverse—until they're standing again in front of the person they love, in the moment when the misunderstanding they are now caught in began.

I was thirty-four years old, standing in my dad's hospital room. But now I'm seventeen years old, in the moment our misunderstanding begins. I am a high school senior who has just decided to play basketball at the University of Colorado, 1,832 miles from home, and it has not occurred to me that my dad—who has taught me the game, who has picked me first in every pickup game we've ever played, with whom I've spent more time than anyone else— feels discarded by my decision, which in turn makes him question how much I valued him to begin with.

The irony is that the moment of misunderstanding begins because we are blind to the main way we are *not alike*. My desire to move on, move away, has nothing to do with my dad and everything to do with my mom. Like her, I was born with a severe case of wanderlust. Staying in the town in which I grew up inspired only one feeling: claustrophobia. If my dad peered over a fence, he'd likely perceive that the grass on the other side was similar to the grass he was standing on, whereas I would be like, "Holy shit, look how green that grass is," then take off running toward it. My mom's thirst for adventure helped balance my dad's steadfast practicality. I was aware of none of this. And in the cruelty of youth, I didn't even plug in "Dad" as a variable in my decision-making process. He noticed, and he was hurt.

There we are, in 1999: a seventeen-year-old with her eyes on the horizon, on the University of Colorado, and a forty-three-year-old who wants more time near his daughter. And this is when the ways in which we *are alike* activate, setting us on a course neither desires. We are both incredibly sensitive but act tough; we both have a long memory for slights; and we both believe our ideas are superior, which should be distinguished from having the same ideas. We rarely saw things the same way, yet neither of us could be convinced to see the other's viewpoint. It was as if years of playing one-on-one taught us we should always be in competition.

A few years after I left for Colorado, our relationship still not recovered, I came out as gay. I specifically told only my mom, which forced her to come out, on my behalf, to my dad. In the ensuing decade, I could never decode what he was actually upset about: that I was gay, or that I hadn't trusted him enough to tell him. And over the years, if the conversation turned to my coming-out process, he'd say, "Kate never actually came out to me," and the hurt in his voice was inescapable.

A sense of preservation motivated my behavior, my reticence to come out to my dad. But it wasn't just *self*-preservation; I also truly believed I was safeguarding the beauty of our relationship, the purity of our shared connection with the game. Nothing had ever tarnished it. My dad had never projected himself onto my dreams, and the only thing that had ever disturbed our equilibrium was my petulance at so frequently losing to him when we played one-on-one.

Back then, when I played women's college basketball, I thought being gay was a failing. I no longer believe this. But during that time, I came to understand that some people saw gayness as a by-product of the experience. It was one of those ridiculous ideas that circulated around female athletes—that playing sports made them gay. For dads in the 1990s, a shadow still existed: the notion that in some way they were transgressing by supporting the athletic ambitions of their young girls. Today I realize how dangerous all these ideas are, but at the time I just couldn't stomach facing any conversation about sexuality. So many dads came to believe that queerness was the cost of having allowed their young girls into the same spaces as the boys—that, in fact, it was *these spaces* that had made them gay.

Mostly, I didn't tell my dad because I was terrible at appearing vulnerable around him. But I was also terrified of sitting with him and hearing him speculate about whether or not he should have let me play at all. (I couldn't fathom that he'd say this, but I'd heard the horror stories from others and projected them onto him.) But imagining him saying this, his willingness to erase the memories and do it all over again without me by his side, just so I wouldn't be who I'd become—I couldn't risk such a moment.

My solution was to say nothing to him, to cut him out of that part of my life. I told myself it would sort itself out, and eventually it did, but what I betrayed with this decision was his trust. For years and years afterward, I knew he was looking at me, always wondering how much of the story I'd left out. Whether I'd left it out for his sake or my own, did it really matter?

Still, when I think of that long-ago moment when misunderstanding begins, I think also of my parents dropping me off at college in 1999. I would be so far from them: a four-hour flight, a twenty-seven-hour drive. We say the usual goodbyes, and I sit on the front steps of a campus building and watch their rental car pull away. The building is on top of a hill, and their car is halfway down when it screeches to a halt. My dad's door opens and he comes back, wraps me in a hug, and says, "I love you so much."

Why did I not say, right then, "Daddy, I'm so sorry I hurt your feelings going so far away. It's not because I don't love you, it's because I have Mom's adventurous streak. I still want to share this experience with you, and I had the most amazing childhood by your side." Why didn't I say that? Because if I did, I'd have nothing later to regret, and regret is a wormhole into the past. I find myself clinging to my regrets, even constructing new ones—mainlining my dad.

I had just crossed the ocean in reverse, then returned to the present moment, and I was staring at him, in his hospital gown, fresh out of surgery, without an answer to his question about whether being too much alike had bogged us down. The idea of our being alike wasn't new to me; his acknowledgment that our relationship had gotten bogged down was. For years I'd wondered if he too felt the unspoken failings between us.

Occasionally, over the years, I would imagine an alternate world where the two of us talked openly about my decision to go so far away to college, where we really listened and understood each other. In the ensuing years in that alternate world, I linger longer in his hugs, I never silence his calls, I don't challenge every opinion he has, I make more time for the father-daughter adventures we'd once had.

I'd snap myself out of these daydreams, convince myself we were fine, that I was overthinking things. But now here he was, doped up on some kind of opioid, confirming that he knew it, too: We were meant to be more.

Why weren't we more?

I looked at my mom, but she had no explanation for me. Kathryn could sense I was having a moment. She squeezed my hand. But nobody could answer my dad's question except me. And I didn't know how to begin. So instead I said something empty, like, "Is that the drugs talking?"

We had plenty of time to figure it out, I told myself.

Chapter 7

THE PHONE CALL

I was driving home from ESPN headquarters in Bristol, Connecticut, when my cell phone rang: *Big C's Cell*. On average, my mom and dad called me 2.3 times a day, and often one called seconds after I hung up with the other, unaware of their synchronized timing. It was the middle of September 2016, and I knew my mom and dad had just left a follow-up appointment with the orthopedic surgeon who had performed my dad's neck surgery. I don't remember feeling any sense of unease as I picked up the phone—follow-up appointments, until that day, had always been routine.

I'd like now to hit Pause on this moment before my phone rings, parachute into the passenger seat, and observe. What ideas, thoughts, and feelings were monopolizing my mind on the first hour of my drive to Brooklyn? They were almost certainly centered around work. I was probably letting myself bob along on a current of ESPN rumors and drama. Working at ESPN—perhaps like working at most big companies—had molded me. I had morphed from a sophisticated organism capable of living across environments to one adapted solely for advancing in the ESPN ecosystem. I was thirty-five years old, and I'd spent the previous six years of my life navigating ESPN's internal politics.

Like most people who worked at ESPN, I was obsessed with the company. It was the kind of place that consumed you, body and soul. When I wasn't at work at ESPN, I was likely getting lunch or drinks with friends who also worked there, and we'd spend hours deconstructing the culture and our futures at the company. The place inadvertently (I *think*, anyway) fostered paranoia; somehow everyone I knew felt they were highly valued and also that their contract was not likely to be renewed.

I'd joined ESPN from the *Philadelphia Inquirer* in 2011 as a writer for their women's brand, espnW, specifically to help with a company-wide initiative celebrating the fortieth anniversary of Title IX. For the first few years, I just wrote—for espnW and for *ESPN The Magazine*. But then, in the aftermath of the NFL's domestic violence scandal, ESPN realized it needed more female voices on its programming, and not just as hosts to tee up men. Even though I had no desire to be on camera, I soon realized that the more TV I did, the more valuable I was to the company.

What I was desperately searching for at ESPN was a way to set myself apart, to make myself distinctive across their massive network without having to continue selling myself as a "personality." It felt impossible. But I was determined to keep climbing the ESPN ladder, because how could I get off it? Career ladders can be like this. Even if the one we find ourselves on is wobbly, or leading us someplace we're not sure we want to go, it usually feels better than starting at the bottom of another one. Also, I was under no illusion that the platform ESPN provided could be easily replicated.

On the afternoon of this phone call, I was likely considering what emails I could send, who I could connect with to help me make my next move within the company. Did I want my own TV show? Not particularly, although that was a silly answer, wasn't it? Everyone should want their own TV show! Did I want a radio show? Also no, though a radio show could lead to a TV show, so—yes, I guess. Did I want to write more? Definitely, but doing TV shows like *Around the Horn* and *Outside the Lines* earned more money and relevance— commodities I didn't know I wanted until I had them.

I did not like my job so much as I was addicted to the tangential benefits of it. I had long sensed I was approaching the moment when these two things—my well-being and my addiction to money and relevance—would be inseparable. I think they call that "selling out," and once I was on the back end of that metamorphosis, my brain would cannibalize my former idealistic self. Yet I changed nothing. Just kept saying yes to TV appearances, kept cashing checks, kept ignoring the voice telling me I'd long ago veered from my intended path.

"Hey, Dad, how'd it go?" I asked. Right away, I could hear the background noise; we must be on the car speakerphone. Mom chimed in—"Hi, Kate, Mom's here, too"—alerting me to her presence.

I knew that the weakness in my dad's left hand, which the neck surgery was supposed to fix, had persisted. Even so, my dad hadn't again mentioned what the neurologist had said before the surgery, about ALS as another possibility. Why would he? Hearing that was scary enough the first time. We all just continued our magical thinking: *Dad's neck? Eh, well, maybe it just needed a little more time to heal.*

When I was a kid, my dad played in a league with a young guy who was diagnosed with ALS. One night, a year after his teammate's diagnosis, my dad and I and several other teammates collected him so he could watch a game. From then on, whenever I read or heard about ALS, my mind flashed to an image: my dad and his teammates struggling to maneuver their friend's wheelchair up the stairs and into the gym.

And since the neck surgery, the idea that my dad almost had ALS, but didn't, had lodged itself somewhere in my ribs. It didn't exist in a vital organ, but if I concentrated, I could feel it lurking in there— something dangerous had been identified and lingered in the air, even if I hadn't seen it myself. At the same time I had this idea that our luck had run out. And our family, we'd had a run of it: good health, accident free, general happiness, financial stability. I couldn't shake the feeling that this thing, this ALS, would become our great equalizer.

"We just left the appointment with my surgeon," came my dad's voice. "He didn't have any good news, let's just put it that way."

"Okay," I said tentatively. "Exactly what did he say?"

"He said there's nothing more he can do to help, that given everything he sees, with the weakness in my hand continuing, that it's his opinion that I have a disease 'in the ALS family'—that's what he said, pretty much matter-of-fact."

"Jerk," my mom cut in, her voice reflecting more fear than I think she recognized. "How can he possibly know? How can he give that diagnosis? There are so many other things this can be. I mean, right, hon?"

"I have more injuries from basketball than I think this guy realizes, and any number of them could be causing this," he said. "But we just wanted to call and give you the update, as grim as it sounds."

"Well, what now? I mean, what's the plan?"

"I'm going to make a call to my primary care doc, and we'll go from there," he said. "But don't worry, this isn't something we need you worrying about, okay?"

"Yeah, okay," I lied, feeling the small knowing that had stayed hidden in my ribs bloom inside my body.

This was the first time we'd been in this position, with a legitimate health scare, so we were in uncharted territory. I asked if they had called Ryan, and they said they were calling her next.

That weekend, with my mom away for work, I drove upstate to be with my dad. He had this habit of doing push-ups and abs during commercial breaks of games, but that weekend he upped the ante. He brought down a twenty-pound dumbbell and placed it next to his left side on the couch. Every few minutes he'd crank out a set of curls. I watched him and nodded approvingly. At halftime he got down on the floor and did twenty-five push-ups. He looked up at me, his chest heaving, and said, "Does that look like someone who has ALS?"

Only one answer existed—*Fuck, no, it doesn't*—even though the accurate answer was that if my dad's muscles, including his lungs and heart, were only in the opening stages of shutting down, then his current physical strength was irrelevant. Of course, I didn't apply that logic, and neither did he—at least not out loud.

My dad kept playing hoops, even as the function in his left hand and arm continued to deteriorate, and I'd anxiously await his call to find out how he'd played, as if a good night on the court might mean the doctor was wrong. Obviously, if you're dominating the local pickup game, you also don't have ALS.

One side effect of his diagnosis, discovered that weekend we spent together, was that I finally started listening to podcasts. That first evening I said good night to him around midnight and climbed into my old bed. I spent the first hour on the internet, researching information about ALS (100 percent fatal, no effective treatments) and reading first-person accounts. Armed with my dad's info—fifty-nine years old, ex-athlete, weakness in left hand, failed neck surgery—I hunted for another disease that could account for his symptoms. Nothing fit. I found one disease, extremely rare, that stayed confined to a single limb, eventually rendering the arm useless but never progressing further. But that disease had only ever been found in young men from Malaysia.

On the flip side, I found dozens of stories eerily similar to my dad's: former athletes or members of the military, onset in one limb, originally misdiagnosed as a neck issue. The more I read, the less I could convince myself that my dad was suffering from something else. My body responded with adrenaline, that special nervousness that feels like your heart is trying to rise from your body.

I snapped shut the computer and lowered it to the floor. Without the light from the screen, the room was dark. I'd been tired, but now I wasn't. At first I tried to sleep, but my mind was processing too much. Was everything I read about—locked-in syndrome, the loss of voice, the eventual shutting down of breathing muscles— really going to happen to my dad? Had he been reading these same things? If so, what was going through his mind right now, in the adjacent room?

My eyes popped open. I reached for my phone and rummaged through my backpack for my earbuds. First I tried music—the new Adele album—but soon her words drifted to the back of my mind, my thoughts again to the front. I needed something that would hijack my brain and force me to focus. And so for the next month, until my body acclimated to the waves of panic it had been forced to process, I could only fall asleep wearing my headphones, listening to a podcast, my mind finally surrendering to intricate storytelling.

The threat of death—your own or your loved one's—has clarifying power. Suddenly the shoddy scaffolding that propped up my career decision making (money is freedom, relevance is power, TV is king) crumbled around me. But after this burst of lucidity, you still must find the courage to act, to rearrange your life. And that's actually the hard part. After the idea of ALS was introduced into our lives, I tried to be more honest with myself about what I wanted from my career, and I tried my best to shape a life within ESPN's walls that felt more meaningful. For years, I spent hours a day cultivating an opinion on, for example, whether the Buffalo Bills were over- or underrated—an opinion that disappeared into the ether the moment after I offered it. At times this made me feel like a day trader, just pushing money around, creating nothing, contributing nothing of lasting value.

After my dad's initial diagnosis, I stopped doing talk radio, a format in which I was forced to dish a slew of empty opinions, and scaled back my appearances on *Around the Horn;* I reengaged with my former editors so I could write more, and focused on *Outside the Lines,* which covered more substantive topics that aimed to expose wrongdoing in sports.

The selfish part of me recognized my dad's disease as an opportunity. Armed with this awful kernel of news—*My dad has ALS*— I could if nothing else at least reshape my existence within ESPN. After six years of saying yes to every request—filling in on Christmas Day, traveling over Thanksgiving—I could finally say no without guilt. I told myself it was about my dad and spending time with him, but sometimes it was just a get-out-of-jail-free card.

Perhaps I'm a master manipulator, but when I'm being kind to myself, I assume I'm just human and that others have used disease as a kind of leverage for themselves, to bring about change they've been too weak to implement on their own. Yet even possessing this terrible magic wand, I could never find the life I needed at ESPN— somehow I seemed never to be where I needed to be, my heart never in sync with my mind.

It took me two more years to finally walk away.

Chapter 8

FUCK YOU, ALS

To say our family was only facing ALS would be naïve. We already had, within our circle, the same bullshit that plagues every family: wounds from long-ago fights, smarting over who calls whom more often, nitpicking annoyances, and on and on. Except that now, with those three letters in our life—A, L, S—we couldn't keep kicking the can down the road. Now we were on a condensed timeline, though just how condensed we could not know.

Even before ALS, I'd find myself wondering when I was going to get around to restoring my relationship with my dad. The diagnosis jarred me into looking at my life, what I'd prioritized, and also at the glass walls I'd built between me and the people I loved the most. Was I willing to let my dad die without breaking through that wall? In a vacuum, the answer was easy: of course not.

So, the obstacle was not just ALS; the obstacle was the calcification of my habits around my dad. I was deathly afraid of being vulnerable around him—the thought of it literally made my teeth chatter—and over the previous fifteen years, we'd developed a style of interaction that allowed both of us to stay in our comfort zones. We talked about sports. We checked in with each other about the day-to-day. We told stories of the past. We teased each other. Vulnerability, it seems to me, needs to be practiced, just like any other skill. The idea that I could just, out of nowhere, lay myself bare to my dad, and he to me, seemed like the kind of wishful thinking that keeps relationships static. Daydreaming about the one transcendent moment instead of making the small changes that actually chip away at the wall.

I realized I couldn't fix our relationship in one dramatic conversation. My dad did not parent me by showing up on Saturdays with expensive presents. He did so by building daily, steady trust until his presence felt as reliable as air. I knew I needed time with him. I needed to practice different habits: touching him longer, looking him in the eye, expressing genuine feelings, dipping a toe into vulnerability. But was I willing to make the changes to my life that would allow me the time and space to make this happen?

Still, at the center of everything was Lou Gehrig's disease, an ailment that has had plenty of moments in the public eye. To name a few: the physicist Stephen Hawking famously lived with the disease for more than fifty years; Morrie Schwartz, of *Tuesdays with Morrie*, died from it; and in the summer of 2014, before my dad was diagnosed, the Ice Bucket challenge, meant to raise money for ALS, went viral around the world.

Yet widespread understanding of ALS remains elusive. Most people still don't know that ALS is 100 percent fatal, and that most people die within two to five years after onset. The disease's spread is relentless, one muscle after another shutting down, until a person is trapped—mind still sharp—in their body. (Among the body's muscles are the vocal cords, the tongue, the swallowing mechanism, the lungs, and, eventually, the heart.) And very few people know how expensive the disease becomes if one attempts to live with it. There's no cure, and there are no effective treatments. Perhaps the most soothing balm after an ALS diagnosis is denial, which my dad employed for a very, very long time, ignoring his body's persistent muscle twitching, a telltale sign of the disease.

My dad's diagnosis hit our family like a blown tire. We'd been cruising along, then—*bam!*—panic as the car starts shaking, quickly pulling onto the shoulder, reassuring one another we're okay, assessing the damage. But we weren't okay. Nothing was working as it had been. And when we pulled back onto the road to go find help, we traveled gingerly, everything on the verge of falling apart.

MAKE YOUR LAST DRIBBLE THE HARDEST

F or a few years, the most important item in our lives was a white key card that unlocked the door to Union College's old gym. During these years, we misplaced all sorts of things, but never—not once, not ever—did we mislay the white key card. Better than the golden ticket, this card gained us access to a full-size gymnasium that was almost always empty.

Be still my heart. Like walking into Disney World after hours, a vague loneliness mixed with a low hum of nervous expectation, wondering if you'll be able to fill the place with your own magic. No feeling exists like that of having a gym all to yourself.

It was in this gym that my dad and I spent thousands of hours. Most afternoons could find us playing a few games of one-on-one, both of us dripping sweat, followed by my dad rebounding for me until it was time to go.

One afternoon, when I was about thirteen or fourteen, he noticed that when I tried to shoot off the dribble, I kept having to reach down for the ball, throwing everything off-rhythm. Strange, the simple solutions that elude us when we're in the middle of a complicated maneuver. Even though I needed the ball to bounce higher so I could smoothly begin my shot, it didn't occur to me that I needed to put more effort into that last dribble. Obviously, if I wanted more from the ball, I had to give more to the ball. But that didn't seem so obvious at the time.

My dad walked over, calling for the ball by holding up his palms. I passed it to him.

"You gotta make that last dribble harder," he said. He demonstrated what he meant, taking two regular dribbles to get where he wanted to go, then a last dribble, which he took forcefully, so that the ball bounded back up quicker and he wasn't left reaching down for it when he wanted to be moving up into his shot.

"Ohhhhh," I said, a revelation, as often the simplest things can be. "I've just been dribbling normally."

"Right," he said. "Always make your last dribble the hardest. Really pound the ball into the floor, so it bounces right into your shooting pocket and you're not left reaching for it."

If you want more from the ball, you have to give more to the ball. If you want more from the ball, you have to give more to the ball. *This sentence would actually flash across my mind whenever I played.*

When I stopped playing hoops all the time, I would still think about this piece of advice and apply it in other contexts. Make your last dribble the hardest. Don't leave yourself reaching back, hoping everything works out—make sure you've created the proper momentum for your next move.

Some moments, my dad was telling me, call for more.

Chapter 9

FEEL MY MUSCLE (PART I)

Within our nuclear family, my dad's idiosyncrasies became legendary, eliciting many an eye roll. He would sing in the shower, usually inserting himself ("The Big C") into the lyrics. For example, the chorus of the Bruce Springsteen song "Born to Run" became "Champs like Big C, baby, Big C was born to run"—no matter that the extra syllables threw the song off-balance. Or he'd roll up his dirty socks and toss them at you. If you were seated, they'd land in your lap and you'd fling them off like they were a rat. He was the oldest of six kids, so apparently he'd gotten used to mild forms of torture and to getting away with everything.

My favorite of his eccentricities was when he demanded—yes, demanded—that you check out his biceps. Not a week passed without him calling me over, or stopping me, so I could confirm that his biceps were impressive. He'd grown up during a time when lifting weights wasn't part of basketball training. And when we watched hoops together, sometimes he would wonder how much better he would have been if he'd had modern training methods.

I would walk past where he was sitting on the couch and he'd say, "Feel this muscle," then flex his right arm. I'd pause, wrap my hand around his bicep, and nod as if I was impressed. In retrospect, I imagine he knew he wasn't the strongest guy in the world—he would do some lifting at the gym, push-ups at night—and this was a form of validation. I'm probably overthinking it, though. Most likely he just thought it was funny.

Picture me at our family's Christmas Eve party, dozens of us jammed into a small house, and my dad waving me over from across the room. I join him, leaning into his side, letting him drape his arm across my shoulder. Then imagine him sweeping his other arm in front of me, balling his fist: "Go on, feel that—feel that muscle."

I can hear him saying that, still.

Chapter 10

OUT OF LOVE

I wish I possessed the same deep, abiding passion for the game that I know my dad had throughout his life. Some people say we shouldn't want to change anything about ourselves. That every part of us, the strengths and the flaws, makes us who we are. Mostly, I agree. But maybe I wouldn't mind if we could turn the dial, here and there, just to make us more compatible with the people we love most. Because nothing caused more separation between us—not my decision to leave home, not my coming out, not any stupid thing I ever said or did—than my realization that I didn't love basketball, that for me it was a means to an end and not an end in itself.

I'd been injured my freshman season at Colorado, so excused from the grueling workouts and emotional pressure, free to enjoy the benefits of a team without paying the price of admission. But that next season, I quickly spiraled. I didn't want to do any of it, every workout, every practice. Just looking at a basketball filled me with dread. Hating anything is unhealthy, but despising something you once believed you loved is especially demoralizing—shame mixes with confusion when you realize that either you were fooled into loving it or now you're deceiving yourself into hating it. *Which part of my life,* you lie awake wondering, *is the lie?*

That sophomore season, I remember sitting in the empty arena a few hours before one practice and wondering how I could hurt myself just enough to avoid working out but not so much that it would be debilitating. After a few weeks of this, I decided the only solution was to quit the team, give up my scholarship, and go back home. What I would then do with myself, I didn't know, but I'd be fine as long as it didn't involve basketball. There were so many other activities I hadn't explored but wanted to: theater, writing, cooking, reading history.

My dad flew out to Boulder after I told the head coach I was leaving the team. Both of them urged me to reconsider. I realized, as Dad and I sat across from each other at lunch, that this was the first life hurdle I was facing with which he couldn't empathize. He'd loved basketball so much that, for him, the scales were never uneven. What he got out of the game always matched, or surpassed, what he put in. Now here I was, suggesting that for me, the scales were lopsided. The benefit of playing was insufficient to the cost. Over lunch he made it clear that while the decision was mine, he believed I would regret walking away—echoing the words of my head coach.

I heeded their advice. I decided to keep playing, but also began seeing a sports therapist. For me, staying was the right decision, although I can also picture a version of my life in which I stopped playing and joined the school's improv group or wrote for the campus newspaper.

For the next five years basketball remained the centerpiece of my days, but I never felt the same about it. My relationship with the game became transactional: I showed up, I did the work, and in exchange I kept my scholarship and identity as an athlete. It wasn't joy; it was a job, and I never again found myself lingering on the court, just soaking it all in, the way I once had as a little kid. Something had broken inside me, and I could never get it back.

This connection, from head to heart, broke long before I came out as gay. And this fading of enthusiasm, of zeal, for a previously adored endeavor would become a theme in my life. Many of us grow up believing that if we can find our one true passion we'll "never work a day in our life." My dad believed this. For him, that one true thing was the game, and I know he thought it was the same for me. But I wasn't built like him. I came to understand that—as the writer Elizabeth Gilbert has articulated—I'm a hummingbird, not a jackhammer. That is, I can't keep at the same thing, pounding away at it, taking pleasure in the routine and slow progress; I must fly from one venture to the next, staying just long enough to make my mark, thrilling at the variety.

My dad couldn't understand—he couldn't believe it. The game had built us. We were the who and basketball was the what, where, when. The car ride to the gym, the tying of our sneakers, the banter, the postgame analysis, the low fives, the shared language: all these things had always been done with mutual delight. Maybe when I was really young, my dad thought he was doing me—the little kid—a favor, but later on we both knew there was nowhere else the other person would rather be.

Then I had to go and fall out of love (or maybe I'd never been in love?) with the game. At first, the shift was almost imperceptible. I'd veered just a degree or two away from my dad, and I could convince myself that nothing at all had changed. But if I look closely, I can see it: I'm not smiling as much, I want to leave the gym a little earlier, I've less patience for the postgame jawing about who beat whom. I imagine I started resembling someone who's gone into the family business but is secretly daydreaming of backpacking through Europe.

Except it wasn't much of a secret. Once I stopped playing professionally, two years after college, I stopped playing almost entirely. It was a relief. This decision was the opposite of my dad's. He came home from his career overseas and joined every league and pickup game he could find, playing as frequently as he could for the next thirty years. Pretty much the only time I played was with him, and even that I could no longer enjoy. I'm shattered to remember the number of times we actually played together when I was an adult—a small fraction of the times he asked me to play with him. It confuses me still, trying to explain how I felt stepping onto a court, though I imagine anyone who's logged ten thousand hours at anything recognizes the loathing that often grows alongside the dream, like weeds in a flower bed.

To his credit, when it came to basketball, my dad was like a puppy dog: when we did play, he held no grudge about my disappearances, just eagerly grabbed the ball, telling everyone we were going to play *just like the good old days.* And during the evenings afterward, his mood was buoyant, and he'd low five me every time I walked past him and wonder aloud what our all-time, head-to-head record was. Had I won more games, or had he?

"It's gotta be me," he'd say, grinning. "Think about the head start I had when you were a little girl and you couldn't even get your shot off over me!"

His joy twisted the knife in my self-inflicted wound. Why couldn't I change this part of me, turn the dial just a little, go back to loving this thing? But what was hardest about the days we did play together was how, inevitably, my dad believed it was the beginning of our renaissance. He'd call me the next morning and say, "Rematch? Next weekend—I'll come to you."

"We'll figure it out," I'd say, putting him off until the following week, again and again.

Sometimes as much as six months would pass between our games together. Maybe even more. And after a decade, that initial degree or two, that slight veer, created a gulf. Years of missed car rides and sneaker tying and postgame Gatorades—all that time together, penciled into the cosmic calendar but never shared.

One moment plays on a loop in my mind: I'm dripping sweat, walking off the court with my dad, and he sits on the wooden bleachers and gives me a quick low five. I am twelve years old in this memory. And I am fifteen, and nineteen, and twenty-three, and thirty-four. I am a little kid, in awe of him; I am a high schooler, annoyed at him; I'm a grown woman, home briefly from her job at ESPN, impatient with him.

My mind has created an amalgam of this interaction: three decades of father-daughter low fives compressed into a single loop, dense and potent, an emotional black hole threatening to implode my heart. You can imagine how many pickup games we won over the years, how many quick low fives we shared walking to the water fountain between games. But it wasn't only on the court. The low five was his signature move—anywhere and everywhere. If I was walking past him on the couch, or if I'd just climbed into the passenger seat of the car, or for no reason at all, say while walking next to him in the aisle of a grocery store, "Low five" was all he'd say; then, if you missed the cue, he'd add, "Come on, don't leave me hanging."

Such an easy, fluid gesture of camaraderie, of love. He'd offer my sister low fives, and my mom, and my cousins, but I'd always watch the rhythm of their palms, and they were never quite in sync. I told myself that a good low five takes coordination, athleticism, and therefore the best of them were shared between me and my dad—it was our special connection.

My dad searched for a replacement bond. I can remember us sitting on the deck together, looking at birds—he was an avid birder—and expressing interest in identifying a large specimen perched on a faraway branch. He eagerly handed me his binoculars, and for the next few minutes I flipped through his bird book, looking for the match. He was almost bouncing in his deck chair, giddy at the thought that maybe this could be our next shared pastime, and that night he relayed my discovery—a common red-tailed hawk, but beautiful nonetheless—with enthusiasm.

But he never gave up hope that I would return to the game. He always seemed to believe I was lost, in a dormant period, and that I'd snap out of it if he waited long enough.

My wife and I now live next to two outdoor basketball courts. A few times a day we drive by them, and I often walk past them, too. I'm always looking for this one kid. By now, he's probably twelve or thirteen years old, though when I first spotted him, he was likely around nine or ten. He's sinewy, with floppy sandy brown hair, and he looks like he's about to hit a growth spurt. Kathryn thinks I'm a little obsessed with this kid, and the truth is, I might be. But I'm obsessed with him mostly on my dad's behalf. The first time I saw him—I don't know his name; we've never spoken—he was alone on the court and he looked peaceful. He was dribbling, and I immediately noticed he had the ball on a string, adept in a way most kids aren't. His shot, too, was smooth and pure, and I could just imagine my dad craning his neck as we passed, hoping to glimpse another skill, pleased at the kid's dedication.

Because, boy, is he dedicated. I see him in the rain, in the heat, in the cold. He's often alone. I feel a kinship with him, having been like him once, practicing everything I saw on TV until the movement was mine. And I also feel a sense of duty, to respect and honor his basketball dream, in the way I know my dad would. But most of all, I'm made aware that the way we each notice the world is unique.

Some cities and towns are built outward from a square or city hall, visitors naturally drawn inward as in a web. But that's never quite how my dad and I experienced new places. Instead, my dad would catch sight of a blacktop or a gleaming hoop down some side street and make a quick turn, taking us into the heart of a neighborhood—into a very different city center.

He could sense the presence of a basketball court from blocks away, the way the streets opened up, and he never missed an opportunity to scout the quality of the rims, the players in the area. The amount of information that could be gleaned, instantly, from a town's basketball courts was not lost on me. My dad would slowly drive by and we'd both get the full download: Cotton or metal nets? Single or double rims? And what were the guys wearing? What color was the court?

I imagine an architect could glance at a building and notice a thousand minor details, whereas I'd notice just a few. Similarly, I can glance at a pickup game and within seconds write a novel about the place and its characters. I know that if a guy is wearing an NBA jersey, he's not very good, and one dribble tells me if someone has any skill at all. In every town we'd cruise by their court, and my dad and I didn't even need to exchange notes. Nothing was in doubt. We'd seen the same clues and they always meant the same things, and we'd look at each other and drive away.

In my neighborhood now, my guess is that a few hundred people pass the courts as frequently as I do, and I'd be surprised if more than a couple have registered the dedication and potential greatness of this boy. What do the rest of them see, in those moments as they drive past those hoops? Some may barely observe the courts at all, in the same way I might not notice a well-tended garden, having never tended one myself. If they don't see this kid, which to me seems impossible since he burns so bright, imagine all the stunning precision and stark beauty I must be missing elsewhere, in places I don't understand. I could be looking right past a masterpiece, if it's from a world I'm unfamiliar with—perhaps as unfamiliar as basketball is to my neighbors.

This young boy moves in a language I fluently speak, and each time I see him, I look for what new words he's carved into the court.

ALWAYS FIND
THE CENTER MARK

O n every basketball court, on the free throw line, there's a small notch that marks the precise center point of that line, from which you can draw a straight line to the middle of the rim. This fact is a piece of trivia that at once seems pointless and also terribly vital, calling to mind blueprints and soaring cathedrals and the third eye and the mathematics that rules the entire universe.

My dad showed me this mark for the first time when I was a little kid. He was standing at the free throw line and he said, "Come here for a sec, I want to show you something." He toed the line—"You see that little notch right there?"—and I knelt down and ran my fingers over the small indentation. "You can find that mark on every court." He looked up at the rim, back down at the mark, up at the rim. "It shows you where the center is—the center of the line, and also the center of the rim." He scooted his right toe to line up with the mark and bent his knees so his right knee was now also in line. And even though he didn't have the ball, he showed how his right hand was in line with his right elbow, which was in line with his hip, which was in line with his knee, which was in line with the mark.

It would be too much to say that, before this moment, I thought basketball courts were ruled by chaos. That's not quite right. The chaos wasn't in the courts; it was in me. I was young, and although I knew and trusted the hoop in my driveway and a few around town, every new gym I walked into felt foreign—an unexplored land. I'd think, In this part of the world, how far up is their rim? How wide and long are their courts? What are their rules?

I was still kneeling by the tiny pockmark, marveling at its existence, my dad hovering over me. "Wow, okay, so you're saying I can find this same mark on any court . . . in the world? And that everywhere it means the same thing?"

"That's right," *he said.* "Pretty cool, huh?"

From that day forward, the first thing I did upon walking onto a court was to go find the center mark. In a game in which so little was known and almost nothing was predictable—what a teammate was thinking, what an opponent would do—this little mark was always there, an anchor of familiarity against which to orient myself.

"When I see this mark, it reminds me to take a deep breath," *he said.* "In the middle of a game, things can feel out of control sometimes. But when you're walking to the free throw line, maybe you're tired, you're breathing heavy . . . that's when you look down, find the mark, get everything in line—get calm."

It's impossible to say how many times—on the court and off—I have thought of this center mark and how my dad was right: I really could always find it, or, later in life, some steady point just like it, amid the noise. For years, I'd forget the calming power of this constant, then suddenly I'd remember.

Marks like these are everywhere, if you know how to look for them. And finding one in the chaos reminds me to breathe deeply and remember that the information I need is already inside me.

My body is in line with the rim, in line with the universe.

PART

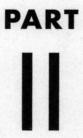

Chapter 11

KATHRYN
(PART I: WINTER 2018)

Occasionally, in the first year after I moved down to Charleston, this thing would happen where I'm with Kathryn, we are out for a walk or in the car, and I'm using the word *home*, except I'm not using it to refer to our home, the one we've built together, but my parents' home—my childhood home. I'll be in the middle of speaking when I recognize that my internal compass for "home" still points toward the house I grew up in, and then I'll panic that I've just confirmed this view with my choice of language, so I course-correct in mid-thought, adding something like, "Well, not my home-home, but my childhood home, is what I mean." Then I carry on hoping she hasn't noticed. Even if Kathryn is gracious enough to let it slide, my insides get all twisted as I quickly do a self-assessment: Why do I still feel that my parents' house is home? Does this mean I'm not really an adult? Am I capable of prioritizing the family I'm creating over the one I came from? Will I ever feel that same sense of *home*?

This particular mindfuck is of my own making—kind of. In our relationship, we've talked about the word *home,* and Kathryn agrees how difficult it is to dissociate that word from childhood. But that's the only overlap between our perspectives on family that I can point to. I know for certain that she wouldn't prioritize her nuclear family over me, and I know this deeply. I also know that she wouldn't say the same about me. The number of times she's been included on a "Fagan family" text chain, then stepped away from her phone for an hour, returning to, say, thirty-seven missed messages, is too numerous to count. She is generous in her response. *Oh, you Fagans,* she'll say, but I know her inner monologue includes very different language.

She wonders frequently about my priorities, where she falls in the pecking order. We could manage if this was a question of my sense of duty—familial obligations, and so forth—but the truth is that her concern cuts deeper. She worries I'm a little obsessed with my family; that maybe the love I siphon off for them bleeds me dry. Half of her apprehension is justified, half fueled by jealousy and sadness over which I have no control. She's jealous not just because she senses that a part of my heart and attention will always be drifting toward home (that word again!), but because she observed my relationship with my dad, our shared history, and she craved the same.

On more than one occasion, Kathryn suggested that the core of our issue was my belief that my dad was more important than her dad. To which I would respond, "That's not true!" Because, well, what choice did I have? How could something like that be real? It could be true in my head—and, I'm embarrassed to say, it was—but it could never be something I said.

In marriage, I've realized that whenever I answer, reflexively and emphatically, "That's not true!" when my wife suggests the existence of a dynamic...it is, in fact, true. I think Kathryn became frustrated at my reluctance to speak plainly about how I viewed our dads. I was always trying to say the "right" thing instead of the true thing, which probably made her feel crazy.

When I thought of our two fathers and the strange competition we'd thrust them into, the song "Cat's in the Cradle," by Harry Chapin, would play in my mind. We'd had the CD when I was growing up, and so I knew every word. It's a folksy tale of a father who doesn't make time for his son, who in turn, when he grows up, doesn't make time for his aging father. The song made me believe that the whole thing was a simple matter of math: you get out what you put in. Kathryn grew up with a brilliant, successful man as her father—he just didn't spend much time with her. Couldn't she see that it was natural—evolutionarily sound, in fact—that the dividends she would pay to her dad would be a fraction of what I'd pay to mine?

(I realize that thoughts like these are what made the dynamic worse, since none of this stuff is actually quantifiable, but this was part of my inner monologue, which she could understand by my actions.)

What Kathryn didn't know is that when I thought of "Cat's in the Cradle" as it pertained to my dad, I felt like a failure, like I was the antagonist in a paradoxical version of the song where the father pours his heart and soul into his kid and the kid is like, "See ya! I'm moving down south while you die!" The dynamic with our fathers began before my dad's diagnosis of ALS and her dad's diagnosis of liver cirrhosis. Back when everyone was healthy, it felt quaint. Not pressing at all. She'd occasionally smile her secret smile when my dad called for the second time on a given day, and I'd say, "What?" like I didn't already know.

Once our choices seemed to have life-or-death consequences, the stakes ratcheted up, a vague kind of tribalism started bubbling to the surface. At least, that's how it felt for me. Intellectually, I understood that I needed to defend my relationship first and foremost, but I would have an almost physical reaction if I didn't show up for my tribe of origin. It's only a slight exaggeration to say that when too much time passed between my visits home, I was riddled with the kind of guilt one might feel watching a raiding party attack the village they've just abandoned. This guilt devoured me for the first two years of my dad's illness. When he was diagnosed, Kathryn and I were living in New York City, about a three-hour drive from my hometown. Getting in and out of the city was a chore, and we saw my parents no more frequently than if we lived a plane ride away.

About the same time as my dad's diagnosis, Kathryn and I had decided we needed to leave New York. Kathryn still owned her house in Charleston, where her parents retired and still lived, and even though that was the most sensible move for us, I struggled with how to position this decision to my family: *Yes, we've just heard Dad has a terminal illness, but I've decided to move farther away.*

At one point, to assuage my guilt, I floated the idea to my mom that Kathryn and I could also get a place near Albany. Maybe we could split our time? A few weeks later, after my mom had had a little too much wine, she got teary-eyed about everything that was happening with Dad, and said, "But you know Dad, all he cares about is spending time with you, and the fact that you've prioritized him means everything to him."

Except that I hadn't. We left New York for Charleston. My workaround included promising that I would come see them every week. I was still working at ESPN, and every Friday I appeared on *Outside the Lines,* which is filmed in Bristol, Connecticut. My plan was to fly up a day early or stay a day later—every single week. I believed I could make it all work: my relationship, my job at ESPN, time with my dad, a life in Charleston. For the first couple of weeks, I tried to do it all, but it turns out that ESPN headquarters aren't all that close to Albany (a three-hour drive), that there are no direct flights between Charleston and Albany or Charleston and Hartford, and that in order to see my parents and appear on TV, I needed to be away from home three days of the week.

Pretty soon, and for the next six months or so, I essentially eliminated the visits to see my parents. At that time, leaving my job at ESPN felt like a nonstarter. I'd worked too hard to get there. I felt my life would derail if I left. During this stretch, only my dad knew what was happening inside his body, but he repeatedly told us the ALS wasn't progressing, that it still remained only in his left arm, which allowed me to believe that time was still on my side. From the outside, it appeared that I'd chosen my job and relationship over showing up for my dad. From the inside, it felt like I'd chosen neither. Kathryn would agree. When I was home, the guilt I felt was inescapable. Guilt that, now a plane ride away, I wasn't as available for my job anymore. Guilt that I was failing my dad. I always had one foot on a plane somewhere—mentally as much as physically. All this made me hard to be around; I was barely present in my marriage.

In early January of 2018, everything came to a head. Just after New Year's, the South got hit with a winter storm, dropping a little over five inches of snow on Charleston—the most snow to fall there in almost fifty years. I was scheduled to fly to ESPN and host *Outside the Lines* and appear on *Around the Horn,* but the Charleston airport—in possession of zero plows—could not remove the paltry accumulation of snow from its runways. The airport was shut down for a week.

Along with the snow, a panic attack unlike anything I've experienced descended on me. I could not get to my job—the thing I had mentally prioritized over everything else. I was willing to be a ghost in my marriage, and abandon my dad, all so I could tread water at ESPN, and now I couldn't even get on a plane to do that.

Kathryn pulled me aside and told me I was making myself ill. She believed I needed help. And I agreed.

Chapter 12

WET LEAVES
(SEPTEMBER 2018)

For a little less than two years, the family policy about discussing my dad's diagnosis was muddled. My mom adopted an upbeat attitude and brushed aside any mention of ALS as out of the question. "There's just no way," she'd say. "What are the odds?" My dad followed her lead (or she followed his), saying that he believed something else was more likely responsible for his wasted left arm. Nevertheless, during those first eighteen months of denial I would often watch him when he didn't think I was looking, and it felt like he knew something was terribly wrong. He just couldn't bring himself to say it aloud.

Nothing else accounted for his symptoms, but doctors offered glimmers of hope along the way, so eventually I made the conscious decision to suspend disbelief and hop aboard the "This will stay in his left arm" train. It was easier that way. I could sleep better. And I could justify not making any drastic changes to my life, including staying at ESPN.

The theory that my dad's "version" of ALS, that it might stay in his left arm, was introduced to us during our first visit to the Lou Gehrig Center at Columbia University. It was early October 2016, the appointment was his first with an ALS specialist, and the hope was that they'd send us away with a definitive *this ain't ALS* assessment. I joined my mom and dad at Columbia, terrified. My life to that point hadn't involved many hard moments. The scariest one had been telling my mom I'm gay, which I'd done scrunched in a ball and pulling a beanie over my eyes as if I could disappear beneath the fabric. I didn't think myself capable of sitting in a room and listening to a doctor tell my dad he was going to die horribly.

After my dad completed all the tests, I walked to the waiting room and watched my mom and dad slip into the consultation room to wait for the doctor. I didn't want to be in that office. Not unless a positive outcome could be guaranteed. But just as I settled into my chair, the doctor popped by on the way to the office and encouraged me to join my parents, promising me that everything looked good.

Holy shit, yes! I jumped up and followed him into his office, and I could sense that he'd already alerted my parents that everything looked okay, because my mom seemed relieved. My dad, though, he was still on edge, leaning forward in his chair.

"Okay," the doctor said, opening the tan folder on his desk, scanning the results. "Everything looks strong: the breathing results are normal, the EMG looks solid, muscle reactions are good. At this point, there's no reason to believe you have ALS."

I remember hearing him say this, and even though it didn't map onto reality, I was content to surrender fully to the doctor's verdict. I'd come to believe that our family was due for a twist of bad luck, but in this moment I easily ignored the law of averages and gratefully hurried back under the warm glow of our perpetual good health.

"Let me just do a few more routine tests, then we'll have you out of here," the doctor said, gesturing to an exam table at the back of the room. Surprised, my dad did a double take—he thought the examination complete—and gingerly climbed onto the table. The doctor placed his hand on my dad's thigh and asked him to raise his leg.

"Good," he said, lifting his hand and moving to the other leg. "Okay, now—again."

My dad tried, grimacing with the effort, and the doctor made the sound you never want to hear from a doctor: "Hmmm." My eyes flew to my mom's, and my heart swung like a pendulum.

"Let's try that again," the doctor said, keeping his eyes down, focusing. A moment later came the same sound again, *Hmmm,* and when he lifted his head, he frowned and walked back to his desk.

Few noises in the English language are as complicated as "hmmm." In particular, I've always had a thorny relationship with it because my dad used it whenever he didn't believe something I'd said but didn't think the exchange important enough to continue. It was a way for him to get the last word without the headache of an extended argument. The topic was usually trivial. For example:

Dad: Let's swing by the dry cleaners on the way home.
Me: I think they close at five p.m.
Dad: I thought they stayed open until six on weekdays.
Me: Nope, always closed at five p.m.
Dad: *Hmmm.*

Dad deployed the sound like a grunt, like machine-gun fire, the emphasis heavy on the *h*. As I got older, I would call him out—"What does '*hmmm*' mean?"—and force him to say what he meant. He found it charming at first, then annoying, like I was always trying to pick a fight.

The doctor's *hmmm* was deeply thoughtful, drawn out, the kind of noise you could panic swim inside of. Not at all like my dad's.

We all returned to our chairs, and it was as if a reset button had been hit. The doctor folded his hands on the desk and looked at my dad. He said, "The results of the clinical exam are consistent with ALS."

"The clinical exam?"

"The tests I just performed, the weakness in one side over the other, that's consistent with an ALS diagnosis."

My dad gestured to the folder on the desk. "But what about what you were just saying?"

"ALS is an incredibly difficult disease to diagnose and presents differently in everyone," the doctor said. "You are strong and show no signs of weakness in your breathing, which for some is where it starts. But there's no telling how it might progress, if it might progress, when it might progress. The disease could stay just in your left arm for a decade. And let's hope that it does."

I'd been tricked into a hard moment. A bait and switch. But I suppose that's how much of life happens: arriving instantaneously, before you have the chance to opt out.

My dad had a lot of questions and, once we left the office, a lot of reasons for why one side of his body could present as weaker than the other. Because of the confusion in this initial diagnosis and the vague projections about what might happen next, our family began Operation Not ALS, and we deployed it in earnest for about two years: from this day at Columbia until the fall of 2018, although for each one of us the timeline of realization is probably a little different.

A few weeks before my wedding to Kathryn, in October of 2018, I was home with my parents for a few days after working at ESPN. It was upstate New York, fall, and the weather was wet and cold. One morning, I woke up and the house was empty. That wasn't unusual. My dad wasn't a great sleeper, nor was he great at letting Mom sleep, so the two of them were often up and out early.

I turned on the coffee machine and not a minute later I heard the familiar childhood sound of my dad's car pulling into the driveway. Astounding, the rhythms and nuances we absorb as kids without even knowing. Footfalls on the stairs. Dishes placed in the dishwasher. Tires over driveway gravel. My mom came through the door first, and everything was off. She was quiet but radiating energy, and when she looked at me, she shook her head furtively, as if to convey something before my dad came in. He was moving uneasily up the front walk, his balance perpetually off from his wasted left arm.

"What? What is it?" I asked.

"I had to call the police," she said. "He couldn't get up. I couldn't get him up. He fell, on the path behind the library."

"Dad...fell?"

Just then he came through the door, and I wasn't sure whether I should pretend that I didn't know. He took a few steps into the living room and dropped onto the corner of the couch that had long ago been established as his.

"So, you heard about the big hubbub?" he asked me, much more animated than I'd expected. "Look out *be-low*!" he faux called, mocking himself.

"What happened?" I sat adjacent to him on the sectional.

"Anybody would have fallen. Seriously. It was so slippery on those leaves and on the wooden walkway. It was the perfect storm—no traction. We'll go back later today so you can see." He used his right hand to lift his left one into his lap, then twisted his mouth and started biting the inside of his lip.

"I mean, yeah, I get that," I said. "Rain makes wood really slippery, then add a layer of leaves—yikes."

My mom walked into the living room. "I was waiting in the car, but thankfully I heard Dad yell for me from the trail. I tried to get him up—we tried, right, hon?—but I had to run to get the police. I was gonna call, but the station is just across the street."

My stomach dropped again. My mom couldn't help him up? All my life, I'd had two specific scenarios that, if ruminated on, would cause a deep emotional ache that made me squirm. The first was the birthday party of a child for which no one shows up. The second was when an older person falls, and with that descent they recognize their impending mortality, the lushness of youth having instantly decayed around them.

"The EMT, he got me up," my dad said. "Even he had trouble because of how wet and slippery everything was."

But my mind couldn't yet jump to the conclusion of the story; it was stuck on those middle few minutes. My mom, on the walking path, tries to help my dad. She realizes he's too big for her. She leaves him and runs to get help. And it is these next few minutes, my dad alone on the path, that I want to turn away from, but can't.

What did he do in those minutes? Did he look at the sky, the trees? Did he touch the leaves? Did he pick one up and rub it between his fingers? Did he keep working to get himself upright, or did he let his head drop against the wood and close his eyes and wait? Did he think, in those minutes, *This is it, isn't it? I'm approaching my end.*

I lingered in this quicksand for a moment, then looked again at my dad. His eyes searched mine. The only time I'd ever seen him fall was when I was a kid. We were going to play hoops in the middle of a snowstorm, and as he walked out the front door, an undone lace got snagged in the closing screen door and he went headfirst into a pile of fresh snow. It was the softest fall I'd ever seen, and we laughed for a long time. *Tim-berrrrrrrr,* he had joked back then.

This was nothing like that. From the couch across from me, he made a circle with his neck and grimaced. His head had snapped back against the ground when he'd fallen. I could see he was in more pain than he was letting on.

"You should have called me," I said to my mom, although without conviction. Who's to say I could have helped? I was having enough trouble listening to the story in its retelling.

"I think I hit the back of my head pretty hard." He was still rubbing his neck with his good right hand. "I'm a big guy, that's a long fall."

"Should we get you checked out?"

"No, no, no, let's just chalk this one up to the weather," he said, pausing before adding, "I probably looked pretty funny going down."

Later that night he texted me, Mom, and Ryan a GIF of a cream French bulldog puppy rolling on its back, unable to get up. "Me, this morning," he wrote. I smiled. I appreciated his ability to bring humor to what was a terrifying few minutes, and I sensed he understood that his rationale—slippery wood and wet leaves—didn't hold water. But he wasn't ready to say that the ALS had spread to his right arm.

But my magical thinking had limits. Two years of pretending ALS wasn't a real thing; two years of deploying denial as a superpower; two years after our initial trip to Columbia and I finally realized: the timer had been flipped and the sand was falling fast.

Chapter 13

KATHRYN
(PART II: WINTER 2019)

I left ESPN in December of 2018, two months after I got married, and two months and two weeks after my dad fell on the wet leaves and I realized that his disease was actually not going to wait for me to get my shit together. I believed for too long that I would know when my dad needed me. He would never ask, of course, but I figured it would strike me, a clear-eyed understanding breaking over the horizon.

That never happened. More so it felt like me gradually, slowly, pulling myself out of the spider's web, breaking free of one belief (but my job is *so* important) after another (what will my identity be without it?), until I was finally standing alone, untangled.

I left ESPN to take care of my dad, but not only for that; I left also because my dad's disease crystallized, for me, how out of love I'd fallen—with myself, with my choices, and with the future "me" that I was building. Sometimes, even when the timing is inconvenient, you have to stop and circle back around and fix what's broken. As scared as I was about walking away from a "dream job," I was even more terrified of who I'd become if I didn't challenge myself to be vulnerable with my dad, if I avoided the lessons our relationship could still teach me.

In early November of 2018, ESPN offered me a three-year contract extension. I turned it down. Instead, we set my final day at the company for November 30 of that year. It was a Friday. That day, I was on the weekly show *The Friday Four,* which was part of *Outside the Lines,* and the crew gave me the final sixty seconds of the show for a parting message. Here's what I said: "So, my hero is my dad, and the news peg is that I'm about forty-five seconds away from the end of my ESPN career—the last minute of it. And I'm lucky enough to have this opportunity, and it seemed like the right thing to talk about because those who know my family know it's a very tough time for us right now. My dad played pro basketball overseas, and when he came home, he would play pickup all the time, and I would tag along. When I was twelve—twelve years old!—he started vouching for me to all his hoops guys that I could hoop, then he would pick me first in the games—probably because I passed to him a lot. Then we would get some Riptide Rush Gatorade at Stewart's on the way home. This was like clockwork. And it wasn't until years after college that I even realized that female athletes weren't as respected. So, for all the dads out there raising girls without limitations, I see you. And to my dad: I love you. And I got your back."

My dad loved that I worked at ESPN more than I loved working at ESPN. Whenever I was prepping for an appearance on TV, I'd call him for his opinion on that day's topics—especially if it was baseball, his specialty. When I did a radio show, I looked for ways for him to phone in to the show as a recurring guest. One weekend when I was on air, he called in from Green Bay, where he and my mom had traveled to watch that Sunday's NFL playoff game between the

Packers and the New York Giants. He provided on-the-ground color; my personal correspondent. He enjoyed talking sports so much that sometimes he'd call me after I'd finished three hours on the radio, wanting to continue deconstructing one of the topics, and I'd gently—and occasionally not so gently—remind him that it wasn't as much fun for me as it was for him.

But I think what he loved most about my job at ESPN was how it made me a popular conversation topic around his clients and friends. He would rarely have brought me up on his own—"never boast" being a core tenet—but he never had to. Everyone else would ask about me, or ask if he was related to me, and he would proudly answer. Because of ESPN, he got to talk about me all the time.

"I guess you're not Chris Fagan's daughter anymore," he would joke, his voice filled with pride. "I'm Kate Fagan's father."

Even so, when I explained that I was going to leave the company— although carefully avoiding his disease as a reason—he agreed with my decision. He believed that I'd worked hard enough in life that, if I felt compelled, I could now pursue the abstract concepts of "meaning" and "happiness."

Yet somehow, even after I left ESPN, for the next two months I remained in Charleston. Yes, I had left my job, but I still couldn't figure out how to take the next step and leave Kathryn, and our life, without validating her worst fears: maybe I *would* always prioritize my childhood family over her?

One particular afternoon, we sat sipping frozen drinks at one of our favorite places in town. At first the decision to spend the afternoon together, drinking and talking, felt like genius. We had that nice, happy buzz and the generosity that came with it. Each of us had plenty on our minds: me on my dad and my failure to show up for him; Kathryn on hers and the unpredictable feelings accompanying his illness—emotions I was too preoccupied to comprehend.

Drinking felt like a cheap escape. Also, I hadn't yet realized that you shouldn't try to drown your sorrows because, as they say, *Sorrow can swim.*

After the second drink, the conversation turned dark. I can't remember why, only that it did. In order not to make a spectacle of ourselves—or, *more* of one—we called an Uber. Outside the restaurant we stood apart on the sidewalk, waiting for the car's arrival, and even in this flash of memory, I still cannot find the source of our disagreement. Silently we sat side by side in the back of this stranger's car. We weren't mad; we were seething—each staring out our respective window. The second we pulled up in front of our house, the Uber's door swinging shut behind us, we resumed talking past each other. I don't remember any specific words or specific exchanges until we got to the threshold of our back door.

Kathryn was just inside the house; I was standing on the landing. I don't think either of us slammed a door, but we could have—that was the energy radiating off us. Then Kathryn said something that, we both still agree, was the lowest moment of our marriage. Before then, and afterward, we carefully avoided using words as weapons.

"Do you think no one's ever gone through what you're going through?" she said, her tone sarcastic and rhetorical. "Do you think no one's ever loved their dad as much as you do?"

In truth, when she said this, my first thought was, "No, damnit, I don't think anyone ever has!" But when I sobered up, I realized I didn't just love my dad, I was obsessing over him. Since he'd gotten sick, I'd regressed to my childhood reverence for him. No wonder Kathryn was resentful. I was living inside the movie version of a father-daughter relationship, and who can compete with that? We both created that moment in the mudroom. I didn't allow room in our marriage for her grieving—not for her own dad or for mine. My grief was just too big; it gobbled up all the air. Even worse: I never questioned my right to all this space. Without asking, or even considering the impact, I assumed she would keep showing up for me, and just make her own feelings smaller if there wasn't enough room.

I had started seeing a therapist a few months earlier. But therapy wasn't helpful, because I already understood what I needed: to rearrange my life so that I was spending more time with my dad. I knew I needed to be with him along the way, not just at the very end. What I didn't know was how to implement this solution without damaging my marriage, without Kathryn feeling, once again, that I valued my childhood family over ours. When I was with the therapist, I spent the sessions redirecting the conversation so that we might not land on the inevitable conclusion. Essentially, I was paying someone to *not* gather an insight about me that I already grasped.

It was February, just a little less than a year before my dad would die, and Kathryn and I were both standing just a few feet from the threshold of our back door, where we'd had that horrible exchange just a few weeks earlier.

"I've been thinking about something," she said, and I didn't know what she might say. I don't remember knowing that I needed her to release me, though in retrospect it seems obvious that I did. "I think you need to go spend time with your dad. I'm not sure what the plan should be, but you need to go. Maybe one week there, one week here—something like that. I think it's important. Go. Do it."

I inhaled suddenly and looked at my wife. Her blue eyes were wide, her face expectant. I exhaled slowly, wrapped her in a hug, and whispered into her ear, "Thank you."

From that moment onward, I split my time between Charleston and upstate New York. Kathryn "lent me" to my dad—at least that's how he saw it, because eventually I found out that each time I landed in Albany, he would send my wife a text:

"Thank you for letting me borrow Kate."

Chapter 14

THE WAY WE SLEEP

W e think often of what is genetic between parent and child: eyes, height, bone structure. These traits, written in our DNA, are inescapable. But they are different from what can be passed down. What's coded within our bodies is not always the same as what becomes similar between bodies within the same orbit. We wonder if that one gesture, or vocal tic, or quickness to anger, is genetic or learned.

On January 17, 2019, my mom called 911 and paramedics rushed my dad to the emergency room. He'd had a pulmonary embolism and spent a few days in the ICU. The parts of him that still partially worked—his legs and lungs—had been drained by the experience, and we wondered if it was a blow from which they wouldn't recover. Nevertheless, at the end of January, my dad was still trying to sleep upstairs in his own bed, next to my mom.

For a few weeks after my dad came home, I don't think my mom realized how bad the nights would become. She was blindsided. My dad could still drag himself upstairs, but once in bed he needed to wear an oxygen mask all night. When he was lying flat, his lungs were too weak to supply oxygen to all of his body. He'd lost the use of his left arm and most of his right, and he couldn't roll over on his own or adjust his body or pillows. Approximately every fifteen minutes, for the whole night, my dad would ask for my mom's help rearranging him. Sometimes this meant rolling him over, sometimes moving a blanket, other times readjusting the mask or placing his arm or hand in a new place or at a different angle. Imagine a child meticulously positioning her dolls for a tea party.

One week passed, then another, and finally my mom explained to me what their nights had become. This was their bedroom, their bed, their marriage. Who else could help? My mom believed she should be doing much of the care, but she was losing herself alongside my dad.

So, for a week in February, then again in March, I stayed overnight with my dad while my mom slept down the hall in my childhood bedroom. We all agreed I'd wake her only when my dad needed to pee in the urinal, at which point I would turn around and cover my eyes as if I were a little kid. But otherwise, it was me and my dad. The artificial glow and flickering light of whatever Netflix show we'd put on cut across the bed in which I'd never before slept.

"Katie, can you do me a favor?" he'd ask, his voice weak beneath the mask, and I'd pop up and walk to his side.

"What's our game plan?" I'd say, wondering what variable needed adjusting: the mask, blanket, pillows, arms, legs—all of it? Early in the night I'd have a full tank of gas. He'd smile, recognizing my energy: "Don't worry, I'll wear you down eventually."

"So, here's what we're gonna do," he'd say, making sure to say "we," making sure I understood we were still on the same team. "Roll me over, then put that big pillow under my head, then fold my left arm so my hand rests against my cheek. But make sure the oxygen tube isn't caught underneath me." Check, check, check, check. Then I'd make sure the blanket wasn't pinned beneath him and give his leg a squeeze. I remember the first time I did this, squeeze his leg. In response, he said, "I can feel the love," and henceforth my mission was to elicit as many *I-can-feel-the-love*s as possible.

The nights wore me down, just as they'd done to my mom, just as they were doing to him. He wasn't sleeping. By the small hours, he'd apologize before asking for something: "Katie, I'm so sorry, but could you…"

I wondered, lying there, how badly the urge to move needed to become before he'd call for me. I also noticed how many millions of small movements, tiny adjustments, my own body made in search of comfort, and how none of my clumsy adjustments of him could ever satisfy the intrinsic understanding each body possesses of how its bones want to lay.

Who among us learns the shape another body craves while sleeping? Not the broad strokes—a side or a back, one pillow or two— but the intimate details of where a hand should be placed, how the blanket should drape. I can tell you with confidence that if my dad were still alive, I could arrange him in an approximation of the shape he'd create on his own. This knowledge remains within me.

After the first week with my dad, while on the road for work, I was falling asleep in a hotel room. I stuffed one pillow under my head, tucked another between my knees and let my arm fold, my hand resting across my cheek. I closed my eyes, but only for a second. Suddenly I sat up. My body radiated recognition, like a form of déjà vu triggered from deep inside. The shape my body was making was the same shape I'd made for my dad. Holy shit! I *slept* like my dad.

And now, every night when I fall asleep and I bend my arm so my hand rests on my cheek, I think of him and how alike we are, how his DNA is mine, but more than that. Our bodies tend toward the same shapes. It makes me think of trees, how even two of the same species can spread their branches differently. But my dad and I, even if he was an oak and I was a pine, we'd both stretch for the sun at the same angle.

Months later, when I told him my newfound insight, my mind blown, he said matter-of-factly, "That doesn't surprise me. We've always been very alike, Katie."

Chapter 15

I HATE MYSELF

It was the end of April 2019, and my dad and I went for a ride in his car—just the two of us. I drove, he was in the passenger seat; he had stopped driving at the beginning of December. The day was wet, early spring in upstate New York, the kind of afternoon that would normally have seen him taking a walk along the bike path, binoculars around his neck, eyes scanning the branches for birds.

But there would be no more walks, no head upturned. His legs were too weak for more than a few steps, his neck muscles unable to lift his head. He often looked like he was praying, chin to chest, eyes pressed closed. But I knew he was just seized by pain. Sometimes he asked me to hold up his chin, to relieve the drag on the back of his neck, and when I did this—always surprised at how heavy a head is—he looked momentarily blissful. The car was where my dad felt most normal, which was why we spent so much time there. He could angle his body to find comfort, and for moments here and there, we could pretend everything was fine. At least, I did. I wondered if he could, too.

"What's the longest you can go without remembering you have ALS?" I asked. We'd decided to park the car up above the Mohawk River, near the lock, looking out over the split-level water. He thought about my question for long enough that I assumed he was calculating the time, adding it up.

"Three seconds," he said eventually. "That's probably the longest I've ever gone."

Surely, he's had more of a reprieve than this.

"I can't escape it," he said. "Every millisecond my mind is still trying to send signals to my muscles, and every time that happens, and my hand or leg doesn't respond, I'm living inside the disease. Every time I breathe, I think about my lungs. Every time I swallow, I wonder if I'll choke. Every time I speak, I hear the weakness in my voice."

I flashed to a memory from college, watching *Gladiator* in the theater. That long-ago night I'd been feeling homesick, sorry for my-self, but as I watched the movie, a new feeling took over: gratitude. Things could have been much worse; I could have been waiting to be tossed into an arena with a lion. Odd, the movie *Gladiator* providing me solace. Odder still that I think of it often through the years—a yardstick for how shitty I'm allowed to feel.

I held up my mental ruler to my dad's current situation. Fuck: he loses. If I were him, I think I'd rather be a prisoner turned pseudo-gladiator stumbling into the arena with a wooden sword. He was clearly having similar thoughts, because a couple months later he proposed to us: "Would you rather have ALS or be tossed into a pit with snakes?" He partially wanted to make us laugh, partially wanted us to recognize that he'd been delivered an all-time shitty hand. I asked: "How deep is the pit? Are the snakes venomous?" (He said he'd choose the snakes regardless.)

My dad loved doing things like parking the car and staring out at a river. He could no longer hold a cup of coffee, let alone lift it to his lips, but we'd developed a workaround. We put a straw in the tiny opening in a to-go lid, and I delivered him a sip for each one I took. He would still say, "Oh, that's good," his eyes closed after every swallow as if reminiscing. Perhaps he was imagining a croissant in the other hand. He loved the ends best—that twisted crunch where the most butter pools.

My dad's life was built around simple pleasures, and over the years he found increasing joy and meaning in each one: a decent coffee, a long walk, talking each day to his kids, a drive while listening to the ball game, a good sweat, the Sunday crossword puzzle with my mom. Even as I admired this structure, I seemed incapable of replicating it. Somehow the arrangement of my days, the way I gleaned value, remained outside my control: the copies a book sold, the number of followers on Twitter. I looked at these metrics every day, and they actually constituted my sense of self. This embarrassed me, but I was addicted to this reinforcement cycle, which I'd created, then crawled inside.

What is it like to be him? I thought hundreds of times each day. We were parked high on the riverbank and the water must have been a hundred feet below us. No one could survive the jump, and a queasiness rolled through my body as I imagined jumping anyway.

"How are you feeling?" I asked as we looked out at the water.

"In what way?" he asked.

"I don't know, in general, I guess. What's going on in your mind? How are you feeling about what's happening?"

"What do you think is happening?" he said in a challenging tone, and I heard in his words mostly pain, some denial. What he really meant was: You think I'm dying, don't you? It felt like he hated my euphemisms—*"the thing that is happening to you"*—yet hated even more a straightforward question that left no room for the hope he was still desperate to hold on to. If I'd asked instead, "How are you feeling about dying?" he would have said, his voice soft and scared, "You think I'm...dying?" There was some part of him (how much, though?) that didn't believe it was happening.

We were tiptoeing around words, stripping them of their clarifying power. I slowly rolled my head toward him and said, "Dad." What I was really saying was: we both know what I'm asking.

"I don't like who I am anymore," he said. "I feel like a loser."

My eyes snapped to his. I realized he was being honest. And my throat did that thing where it seizes, my breath catching, as if my body knew better than to let this thought reach my center.

"But you're still you," I said. "How could you ever be a loser?" I felt a little like a kid whose favorite toy had confessed crippling insecurity. I was blindsided that he was even capable of thinking such a thing about himself.

"I'm losing everything that makes me who I am," he said. "I can't do anything that makes me, me. Think about it: I can't do any of the things I used to do to help you. I can't bring Ryan her morning coffee. I can't help Mom. I'm a taker now, a burden. I can't give—I can't give to my family. Life just happens around me, and I can't contribute."

"But those are things you did," I said. "They're not who you are. The disease can't change who you *are*."

"If only it was that simple," he said.

The next day my body was relaxed when his words—*I don't like who I am anymore*—launched a sneak attack, slipping into my heart, and it felt like a sickness spreading inside me. I let myself feel what his words meant, and I was distraught at the revelation: we are never in control, no matter how carefully we plan.

Unlike my life, my dad's was not a high-wire act; he was not seeking fame and relevance and adoration, which can never be held on to. He had found meaning in lifting his head to the trees, walking on paths, bantering with family, holding a coffee. Now these were all gone, save one, and even that would go with his vocal cords in a matter of time.

But the disease also felt personal. My dad, the coolest guy I knew—my *dad*—was being eaten alive. It had already taken so much, it couldn't take his sense of self, too.

I did the only thing I could think of. I sent my dad some words.

Subject: NYC-LA
Date: April 21, 2019, 3:33 PM

Hey, Dad.

How about this? An email from me.

We are currently en route to L.A., but I am thinking of you. I've been thinking, especially, about what you said in the car the other day when we took a drive over to Rexford. You were talking about how you don't feel like yourself anymore, that you feel like a loser (I can't remember if you used that word) because you feel like you aren't useful anymore and can't give and do in the ways that you used to.

That feeling makes sense. I do not know what it's really like to be inside your body right now, no matter how much I try to empathize. And I also can't know what it's like to be inside your mind right now, with everything you're going through.

But I wanted to take a few minutes to tell you a few things. About how who you are has made me who I am. And that nothing—not even malfunctioning neurons—can take that away.

First of all, even right now, you're giving me things and showing me how to be better and how I want to live life. Each time you say, "I can feel the love," you're giving me enough love to make me want to stay awake a hundred nights to be around you. Each time I get a fist bump, you're giving me the same connection that a high five used to. Each time you come up with a witty retort, or joke, you're reminding me that that's how I want to look at life, too. Even when facing the worst of it.

Who you are, right now, is offering so much—even if it doesn't look like it used to look, even if it doesn't look how we want it to look. And I am not suggesting that I wouldn't want to make this all go away instantly because "look at the silver lining" but rather that even in this situation over which we have no control, you are still a person I want to spend as much time with as possible. You are still someone I would choose to be around because of who you are and how you are in the world.

Now, beyond all of that, you have made me who I am. (With Mom's help, of course, but this isn't about her, okay?) You spent your life spending time with me. Every time we walked into a gym together, it was like I was walking in with a god: the best player in the gym. But somehow it was never really about how great you were at basketball, it was about how you always made me feel like I was your teammate. That we were in the thing together. And about how you made sure to create moments that were just ours. I can name so many of them: every time I drive south, through Jersey, and I see restaurants we passed on the way to Giants games; every time I'm wondering where we should go to dinner and I want to rank our options and throw them in a hat; every time I look in the backyard and imagine running routes; every time I drive by a baseball field and I remember the Saratoga duffel bag we had filled with baseballs that you'd toss me; every time I pass a Stewart's—literally, any Stewart's, at any time.

But the thing about walking into a gym with you and feeling proud? It also wasn't 'cause you were tall and strong. It was because you were you, my dad, and you loved me so much and thought I was cool and fun. And I felt safe.

And that's still who I'm with, and how I feel, when I'm with you. Even when we're going into the clinic, I am proud that I am there with you; I am proud that you're my dad.

And as much as I can be in this with you, without truly knowing what you're going through, I am.

Okay. I am now going to watch a movie on this flight.

I love you.

Lesson #4

OCCASIONALLY BANK IN A FREE THROW

*R*yan and I, neither of us could have grown up boastful. Before we learned to walk, we learned not to brag about our walking, and although that's an exaggeration, only barely. One of my dad's core life philosophies was: Don't tell people you're good; let them figure it out for themselves. I heard a version of this hundreds of times. Not because I tested his doctrine—I bought in right away—but because so many other people did. Even at a young age, I recognized bragging of any kind as an unattractive quality. Of course, I'd been primed to feel this way.

My dad could take modesty to extremes. In conversation, he would omit factual details if they sounded too arrogant on his tongue, forcing the other person to ask six questions to gather the information that should have come with just one.

"Oh, you play basketball?" someone might ask, to which my dad would reply, "Yeah, I play a little." Then the person might ask if he played in high school, and my dad would say that yes, he had, but volunteer nothing more. "What about college?" they'd ask next—and on and on. By the time I was in high school, I'd be so bold as to throw my arm around my dad's shoulder and drop his credentials for him: Division I, five years playing in Europe, probably still the best player in the area, and also...my dad—isn't he great?

The unspoken rule: anyone else, even blood relations, were allowed to boast on your behalf.

When I was little, this concept of modesty-as-the-apex-of-character seemed black-and-white. Any words or behavior that fell under the very broad umbrella of "arrogance," including swagger and showing off, I thought were unequivocally off-limits. I did not see nuance. So, imagine my confusion when I was about twelve years old and my dad and I were finishing up in the gym with ten free throws each. Before we started, my dad said, "Whoever makes more gets to pick what's for dinner tonight, how about that?" Those were big stakes in my world. The food was not as intriguing as the idea of control.

I went first and made nine out of ten. I was feeling pretty good; I had a chance. But I knew my dad could easily make all of his. He walked to the free throw line and, without breaking rhythm, made his first nine shots. On his ninth make, I caught the ball as it dropped from the net and tossed it back to him. If he made this shot, he would win.

"There's no chance I miss this one," he said, looking at me, a little smirk pulling on his lips.

"Oh yeah?" I said, having no clue what else to say.

"How about I close my eyes to make it fair? Give you a fighting shot." He squeezed his eyes shut and lifted the ball to shoot. He released the ball with a perfect flick of the wrist, but I could see right away that the ball had too much arch. He'd closed his eyes. That had thrown him off.

But then I watched as the ball came down, kissing gently off the white square of the backboard, then dropping through the rim. I'd never seen anyone bank a free throw, because the board was almost *exclusively used when you were at a side angle. The ball bounced on the ground once, then twice, before I corralled it. I looked at my dad— no change in expression.*

He winked and started walking off the court. Oh, now I see, I thought. He hadn't gotten lucky. He'd purposefully used the backboard; he'd purposefully upped the degree of difficulty. *It was like he had said, without saying,* Keep working, kiddo, you've still got a ways to go.

We started gathering our stuff, getting ready to leave, when I asked, "Why'd you do that—close your eyes and use the backboard?"

"To show you that I could."

"Kinda felt like showing off," I said. "Isn't that like... bragging?"

"Maybe, in some situations," he said. "But even more important is that you don't hide your greatness. You have to let people see it. And sometimes let people see it in full force. You can't make yourself lesser, smaller, just to make people feel better. When you work hard to become great at something, that's your greatness. You own it—not other people."

My growing brain was trying to process this in real time, and I said, "So why did you just bank in the free throw?"

"You tell me," he said. "How did it make you feel?"

"Besides just annoyed at you, I was impressed. It made me feel like there's another level to reach, if I wanted to."

"Well, then, mission accomplished," he said.

"Okay, so the rule is that I can go around... being great, just not going around telling everyone I'm great?"

"That's right: be as great as you can be.*"*

Chapter 16

BACK PORCH

Our family house sits on half an acre of land, or maybe it's a quarter of an acre—I'm not sure. When I was a kid, an acre was huge, like the size of a farm, and even though I now have a general sense of an acre's dimensions, I still feel like the word sounds like more land than it is.

One afternoon I was sitting on the wooden steps of our deck looking at the backyard where I used to run routes. Back then, I was the receiver, my dad the quarterback. He would have the football tucked under his arm and he'd outline the route with his right finger on his open palm, the two of us huddled away from the imaginary defense. Then we'd line up and he'd say, "Blue, forty-two, hut, hut, hike"— always the same call signal—and I'd take off running, mimicking whatever pattern he'd drawn.

That's what I was thinking about—our fall afternoons before Giants games—but I didn't tell my dad, who was sitting next to me, because I wasn't sure if he'd enjoy the memory or feel crushed at the universe so aggressively repossessing it. He was in his motorized wheelchair, which had become necessary that spring. We were facing each other on the stone patio, and he extended his right leg, which he could still move, toward me. I placed my left hand on his shin. His face, once round and full, was now thinner, sallow. His arms dragged on his shoulders, which dragged on his neck, which dragged on his very being.

Even before this disease, I was worried about his aging body. I don't think I'd ever seen him stretch, and he had so many wear-and-tear injuries. Some say ALS is a painless disease, because you don't feel the motor neurons as they die, but that ignores the ripple effects on the body. I'd never seen my dad in so much pain; he hadn't been comfortable in two years.

He was lifting and bending his right leg, which he did frequently, simply because he still could. Then he said, "This would be the best disease to get if at the end they were like—*surprise!*—there's a cure."

"Oh, yeah?" I said, trying to make my voice sound like a casual prompt. Really, I was aching for optimism and this felt something like that, even if it was a make-believe scenario.

"Think about all the lessons I've learned, all the things I've taken for granted over the years," he said. "My god. I could name a million." He started bouncing his leg excitedly, living in this alternate universe where ALS is nothing more than a grueling, immersive life lesson.

He was looking out over the yard, then slowly turned his eyes back to me. He started naming the small things he never recognized before.

"Looking up at the sky."

"Scratching an itch, in the moment the sensation arises."

"Adjusting the waistband on my shorts exactly how I like them."

"Smushing a pillow to the correct depth."

"Carrying my own wallet."

He was purposefully not naming the big stuff—the running and eating and traveling and hugging. I started to think of these small things as the ground layer, the movements so myriad and small we crush them beneath our feet without even looking down. And yet they form the soil from which the more beautiful, elaborate, actions spring. My dad now saw the soil clearly for the first time.

The last small action he named—carrying his own wallet—had come up repeatedly over the previous few months. He'd always been someone with precise locations for his wallet and keys—at home, in the car, at his office. When I was growing up, this eccentricity irked me, because whenever I'd borrow the keys for something, he'd call out, "And make sure you put them back by the phone!" and I'd be like, "Oh my god, the *whole town* knows your keys go back by the phone!" Whenever his wallet or keys went missing, his default instinct was that someone (first Mom, then me, then Ryan) had messed up his system. (He was usually right.)

No longer being responsible for these items hurt him in a way that, at first, I couldn't understand. With everything going on, was this really keeping him up at night? I said something like, "What's the deal with being so upset about Mom having to hold your keys and wallet?"

He thought about my question, then said: "It's like there's nothing that's mine anymore. A wallet, keys, those are so emblematic of a life, of responsibilities, of freedom. Everyone has things that are just theirs, that they're responsible for. Except I don't—not anymore. It's the feeling I miss more than the tangible things."

"Do you think if this really happened, if after years with ALS, at the very end, there was a cure, but not just a cure, a reversal of symptoms so you were restored to exactly how you were at fifty-nine, before diagnosis, do you think that every moment for the rest of your life you'd just be blissfully happy and grateful? Do you think every time you, like, lifted your hand, you'd stare at it in wonderment that it was moving?"

He closed his eyes, took a spin around this imaginary world. "No, I can't imagine that's how it would work," he said. "I think pretty quickly I'd start forgetting about all the small movements, the little things. That stuff would fade to the background. I'd have to make room for living."

I was surprised by his answer, but I saw what he meant. I pictured an overloaded computer, each application running slowly because it's trying to run everything. Similar to his life right then, but inverted: instead of mourning every failed brain–body signal, he'd celebrate every success. That would take up a lot of time.

I thought about what he meant when he said, *I'd have to make room for living,* and I had this flash of awareness. He meant that our brains weren't supposed to recognize every movement our bodies produce. The fact that he did was unnatural. We can't live in that encumbered state. Not if we want our minds free for thinking, or simply for silence. And yet sometimes I behave as if my job is to fill my brain with a steady stream of useless information just to *keep it* from thinking, from silence.

"But the big stuff, oh, man," he said, taking one last lap in his alternate universe. "The runs, the hikes, the hugs, the lifted glass— if suddenly I was cured, I imagine I'd have at least a moment, each time, where I paused and relished the feeling of it."

Lesson #5

LIFE'S MOST IMPORTANT METRIC

When I worked at ESPN, I did a podcast called Hot Takedown *with some guys at Nate Silver's site, 538, which was hyperfocused on analytics. These guys loved finding new ways to quantify a player's, and therefore a team's, effectiveness. Upon first looking at each sport, the starting point was boiling down each game to its most essential metric, then building back up from there.*

For example, in baseball, the most important metrics were runs and outs. Bigger data points, like wins and batting averages, were made up of a whole lot of runs and outs. In some ways, the stuff these guys talked about was like rocket science: they built models, talked about regression to the mean, used complex algorithms. In other ways, it was shockingly simple: look closely at what matters, strip away everything else. Every time I'd go into the office to record the podcast, I'd think about my dad, and how he long ago homed in on the crucial metric for a much more important game: life.

My dad and I went to the Union College gym almost every day, but we did not linger there. From as far back as I could remember, we were focused, and especially so as I got older and the stakes got higher. If I had to guess, I'd say on average we spent an hour in the gym.

At one point when I was about fifteen years old, I started hearing that other players I knew were spending all afternoon in the gym—hours on end. Was I being outworked? I brought this concern to my dad.

I was kneeling, tying my sneaker, and I said, "Maybe we should stay longer today."

"Why is that?" he asked.

"Other people stay in the gym for hours and hours. What if that's what I need to do?"

"What are they doing in the gym for these 'hours and hours'?"

I shrugged. "I don't know."

"So then why do you think you should be doing that?"

"I guess because more time must be...better, somehow."

"It's not about time, it's about attention," he said. "When I was growing up, I'd spend all afternoon at the Boys and Girls Club, and I'd see guys there all day, just drifting around the gym, talking, occasionally dribbling a couple times, walking to the water fountain, maybe taking a couple shots. They'd be there three hours and accomplish a quarter of what I could get done in thirty minutes. Don't be fooled, Katie, you don't get better through osmosis; you can't just spend time somewhere, thinking it'll somehow get into your bones."

I switched feet, started tying the other sneaker. I was relieved. Although I hadn't known it beforehand, this is what I'd hoped he would say. Spending all afternoon in the gym sounded exhausting and claustrophobic.

"This is important," he continued. "Just showing up somewhere, being physically present, is not the same thing as being focused and attentive. If you have the first without the second, what was the point of being there at all?"

Chapter 17

FORT MOULTRIE

There's a narrow street in Charleston—Huger Street—that cuts across upper downtown; Kathryn and I happen to frequently find ourselves there. One of our favorite restaurants is on this street, and it's also around the corner from Hampton Park, where we walk our dogs a few mornings a week.

Kathryn doesn't know this, but the street is haunted. Each time we drive down it, a scene plays out, and sometimes so vividly I have to remind myself it's happening only in my head. (Or is it? Maybe there's also an energetic imprint on the street.) The scene is excruciatingly simple. I'm in the car with my dad. He's driving. It's the night before my wedding—October 3, 2018—and we're driving slowly on Huger looking for street parking. We find a spot, but we need to parallel park, so my dad pulls the car past the opening, lines it up, shifts the car into reverse, and begins to crank the wheel.

I'm looking over my shoulder at his progress when the car suddenly stops. He looks at me, his eyebrows arched, his eyes big. "I need you to do it," he says. "I—I can't, this wheel." His left arm, long rendered useless, dangles from his shoulder; his right arm, the one on which we've pinned our hopes, keeps slipping from the top of the wheel.

"I got this," I say, popping out of the car and darting around, believing the faster I park, the less time my dad has to analyze what just happened. And this is the moment. I see as a drone would, from above: the silver car idled on Huger, both our doors open, me scrambling around the hood, my dad dazed, struggling to pull himself from the driver's seat. I quickly park the car, pretending that the wheel is sticky, grimacing for effect. "Man, that's a really tough steering wheel," I say as I get out of the parked car. It's one of those lies we build to get our hearts from one moment to the next, like grabbing someone's arm and dragging them from a gruesome sight.

Each time we drive down Huger, no matter the time of day, this scene plays. And sometimes as we pass the exact place on the street, I turn my head to keep my eyes there, just to stay in the moment a little longer.

It's no mystery why this has happened. Just hours before he and I drove down Huger, my dad and I had talked—finally talked—about all the failures and miscommunications in our relationship over the years. It was the kind of conversation I promised myself we'd one day have but worried we wouldn't. Nearly a decade had passed between me knowing I had things to say and actually saying them. And for two of those years, my dad had an ALS diagnosis hovering over him, and still I couldn't figure out how to carve out time just for the two of us.

But earlier that day, I'd asked if we could go for a ride, just us. As I knew would happen, my dad's eyes darted to mine, and he said, "Uh oh, am I in trouble?" Now that he was sick, he balked at interactions presented as "special." He thought they meant the other person believed he was dying, and if the other person believed he was dying—well, that was incorrect messaging for the powers that be, the big man upstairs. This kind of reverence for spoken ideas isn't unusual. Many of us believe we can speak things into existence. We think that if we say our hopes aloud, the universe might just conspire to help us. And so, conversely, we worry that if we name our gravest fear, the thing we desperately hope isn't true…well, what will the universe do with *that* energy? (Nothing good, my dad imagined.)

"Let's just spend some time together. I know a cool place," I said, and, giving me another wary look, he accepted.

We drove to Sullivan's Island and parked the car facing the cannons of Fort Moultrie and, just beyond, the expanse of the Atlantic Ocean. The row of war machinery rests between two forts that feel as if they're part of the lush hillside, and along the winding path detailed signs explain the strategic importance of each variation in the landscape. From this perch, with nothing in view but relics of long-ago battles and swaying palm trees, modern life can feel like an abstract concept.

Even in October the temperature was touching ninety degrees, and my dad had his window down. For a few minutes, we said nothing. I shifted in my seat, took in a deep breath. My mind was filled with a jumble of *ums*, *and*s, *I just*s, *I wanted to*s—these false starts, this wheel spinning. Sitting there, finally in the moment I had wanted to create, I was still unable to imagine myself saying the things I needed to say.

For thirty years, our language had been low fives and the New York Knicks and practical advice and sneakers. My dad's love had been expressed verbally through his signature text "aml"—all my love—but mostly through service: he mailed me cards with cash for a dinner out, he drove my car from New York to Colorado, he carried my gym bag around my summer basketball tournaments, he showed up for everything that was important to me. For all this, my gratitude was expressed simply: *Thanks, Dad; you're the best.* We paved over the mistakes and miscommunications and kept chugging along. But what we never did was get in there, wade into the mix of awesome and awful, and see each other clearly.

Sitting next to him, I realized that if I waited for a poetic way to begin the conversation, it would never start. I just needed to dive in and thrash about until I found my footing.

"Um, I just...wanted to get some time together to, to talk, because I feel like there are all these things I want to say that I've never said before—I don't think I've said, anyway."

His eyes turned soft and tender, and he opened his body to me. He could hear the tone of my voice, how it was running along the edge, threatening to fall into the pool of tears below.

"I don't know, I just don't think you realize how important you are to me and how grateful I am...that...you're my dad. I mean, all the time we spent together. How many dads do that? You took me everywhere with you, and you showed me everything you loved, and now I love those things, too."

"I'm not sure I deserve that much credit," he said, putting his right hand on my shoulder. "It wasn't a sacrifice to spend time with you. I really liked you."

"I just always think about all the hours you put in rebounding for me, a little girl, like I was the most important thing in the world. I can't have you thinking I don't remember that, that I don't see that and think about it all the time. That we had such a great childhood and you treated me equally and gave me all these opportunities. I mean, I didn't even realize people thought female athletes and women's sports were inferior until, like, five years ago."

He laughed. "It was so much fun for me, those years, getting to watch you and seeing you fall in love with the game. I had as much fun as you did. Maybe I should be thanking you."

"I'm sorry I went to Colorado without thinking about how it would make you feel. I just didn't, I didn't even think of how it would change everything, and how hard it would be for you to not be a part of that chapter of my life—" and here my voice lost its balance. "I don't think I ever said I'm sorry."

"And you never needed to say you were sorry. Going to Colorado was a great decision for you—haven't I said that, in retrospect?"

I nodded, fat tears falling down my cheeks. Seeing them, he said, "Katie, oh, honey," and touched my hair, and I thought how stubborn I'd been, missing him so much for so long and yet doing nothing about it. I wished I'd said something before the diagnosis, before the clock had started ticking.

"And I just—I'm sorry about how I came out as gay, that I didn't tell you directly, and I'm sorry about that email I wrote when I was mad at you. I'm sorry—I'm sorry I let myself put that anger down in words and sent it to you."

"I made mistakes, too, and I still think about them. I should have come play in that tournament with you in Los Angeles—I regret that to this day. But none of those regrets, or none of our mistakes, changes how much I love you or how proud I am that you're my daughter. I mean, Katie, you've given us so much. I get to be the guy who walks into a room and people want to know if I'm your dad."

"But then you have to tell them you are," I said, trying to make him laugh.

"I am so incredibly proud of who you've become," he said. "And I know it's important to say these things, to talk them out, but you must also know that there's nothing you could say or do that would change the way I feel about you."

And so, hours later, as we were driving down Huger, there was still this kinetic energy between us, this palpable warmth and softness that we'd both missed so much. More than just love, it was a kind of breaking open.

It's this energy, this feeling, that is now trapped in amber alongside the scene—a bird's-eye view of the car, doors open—on that downtown street. And if it's possible to feel a kinship with streets, I do with Huger, because a small part of my dad lives there.

KEEP YOUR SNEAKERS
IN THE TRUNK

One summer when I was ten years old, we vacationed at Bethany Beach, in Delaware. On the first morning, my dad and I went out for a quick drive, to see the downtown, the boardwalk. His eyes lit up as we rolled to a stop sign, and out his window he spotted an outdoor court with what looked to be a competitive pickup game. Guys were even standing on the sidelines, waiting for next.

I was sitting shotgun, peering out the window across him. He was wearing a tank top and shorts, and I watched as his tan arm cranked the wheel, quickly turning us toward the courts, where he parked the car.

"What are we doing?" I asked, unbuckling my seat belt.

"Come on, let's go." He was already out of the car. "Gonna see if I can catch a game."

"But how—you don't have your sneaks." I heard the sound of the trunk popping. "And...we don't have a ball."

I could hear him rummaging in the back. He had this habit of not answering questions right away, making me ask them repeatedly. I got out of the car. The morning was bright, hot, and humid.

"You don't have your sneaks, though," I said again.

"Come on." He shut the trunk and turned to cut across the grass. I could see now that he did, in fact, have a pair of sneakers gripped in his right hand, and so I jogged to catch up with him.

Every few months, all my life, I've had this dream in which I'm meant to be playing in a game, but I can't find my sneakers. Sometimes they're back at my house, which takes me hours to reach; other times they're trapped inside my locker, the code to which I've forgotten. On the rare occasion I find my sneakers, I'm mystified to find the laces removed, or for reasons unknown I spend what feels like hours trying to get them on my feet. In none of these dreams do I make it onto the court.

To be haunted in this specific way, wandering around a sneakerless world, is ironic. Because after this morning in Bethany Beach, once I got old enough, I always put a pair of sneakers (laced!) in my trunk. If you walked out to my car right now and popped the trunk, you'd find a pair of sneakers tucked away, just in case. I can't remember the last time this proved useful, unless you count the smiles and memories the sight of them inspires.

"You just never know when you'll find a game," my dad said that morning.

Too many people let tiny hurdles stand between them and the thing they love doing, the thing that fuels them. The timing's not right, or the guitar's not tuned, or the light's fading. When my dad said to always keep a pair of sneaks in the trunk, he meant it literally. But he also meant that life could sometimes conspire against us, create friction, convince us that doing what we love is a hassle, not a joy.

Our goal is to not let it.

Chapter 18

NOT A BUDDHA

M y dad used to call me anytime someone on ESPN used the phrase "locker room guy," because he thought the phrase had become hollow, deployed mostly by athletes to avoid saying anything real about a teammate who'd, for instance, just tested positive for steroids or gotten arrested.

Example:

Reporter: What's been the response since [so-and-so] was arrested for domestic assault?

Athlete: All I can say is that he's great around the locker room. He's always been a great locker room guy.

"You know what I'm so sick and tired of hearing?" he'd call and say, and I could sense where the conversation was going. "What's it even *mean* anymore if a guy is 'good in the locker room'? Can we stop using this phrase? Katie, can you please tell everyone at ESPN to stop using this phrase? It's a throwaway line so nobody has to actually tell us what they think about someone."

My dad believed our words and descriptions of people should, generally speaking, reflect the actual person. He also wanted that standard applied when others spoke of him. He was terrified—in the days after I published an article about our relationship and his disease in the *Players' Tribune*—when former teammates sang his praises in emails and on social media. *Best teammate ever. Genuinely the best guy in the world. Just so nice—to everyone.*

These notes left him spooked. He was losing control of everything, and now even the authenticity with which people viewed him. Most of his life he'd been the biggest guy in any room, someone you didn't treat with kid gloves. He had walked away from hundreds of basketball courts, leaving a trail of grumbling opponents (and the occasional teammate) in his wake. Sometimes he could be a ball hog; and he also threw vicious looks, and choice words, at more referees than I can count.

But then came ALS and the softening of his edges. Others were rewriting the truth of how he had once moved through the world. Apparently, he told me more than once, he was now someone people needed to pull punches around. It felt like parts of him were being erased while he was still there, like he was a body going up in smoke. He could feel his grasp on who he was—the story of his life—shifting out of his reach.

"It's kind of freaking me out," he said, reading those praising emails. "I always thought I could be a bit of an asshole." (He could be.)

My dad wasn't a philosopher. He was a good husband and the father of two daughters who came of age in the generation after Title IX was passed, a man who loved and respected us, who tried to teach us a belief system and work ethic that would serve us well.

But death, it seems, creates a hero. Flaws are forgotten; mistakes washed away; stories bent to mean something they never did. I'm wary of that. I don't want to create a false standard. Not everyone facing death, in the midst of dying, is devoid of anger and self-pity; if we believe they should be, because that's what we've read in books and seen in movies, we'll become critical when our loved ones don't meet that impossible standard.

I held my dad to that false standard for most of the last year of his life. I regret doing so. I thought he should be like Buddha, or Morrie Schwartz from *Tuesdays with Morrie,* or any number of stoic philosophers who embrace their final days with a pure heart, conviction of the world's oneness flowing from their lips.

When my dad fell short of how I wanted him to act and feel, I couldn't even pretend to hide my disappointment. I'd pounce, say something like, "Is that really a healthy way of thinking about this?" He didn't have the energy to argue with me, something we'd become very good at over the years. He'd play his trump card early—"You can't possibly know what it's like to have ALS"—and sometimes even that didn't slow my judgment of him.

My mom witnessed it more frequently than I did, but in that last year he would thrash in his hospital bed, which was in our living room, repeatedly slamming his right leg against the base of the bed in a fit of anger and sadness. The amount of frustration he could exhibit while having only one working limb was impressive.

He also despised it when people used words such as "journey" to describe dealing with ALS—i.e., "Every ALS patient handles their journey differently"—and upon hearing or reading the term, his face would twist into disgust. He'd say, "Well, if I'm on a 'journey,' what exactly is my destination?" At one point, he saw an interview with an ex-NFL player with ALS on *60 Minutes,* during which the guy said he saw the disease as a blessing and that the years with it had been the most rewarding of his life. My dad didn't feel that way. And he lacked the imagination at that moment to believe that others could be having a fundamentally different experience with the disease than he was. He believed it was a nice thing to say, to try to convince people of, but he couldn't accept it as sincere.

My mom, my sister, and I had dozens of conversations, increasingly so toward the end, about how impossible it was to expand my dad's perspective. To him, everything was judged against having ALS. If you could move your limbs, then your life was still on track. My mom was his full-time caregiver until about the final six months, when she hired Mary Rose, who would help in the morning, and Jeanine, who would come for the bedtime routine. But even so, it was my mom who was always there, who slept on the couch downstairs by his hospital bed, who rarely left the house, who had not slept five uninterrupted hours in a year, and who was so strung out that she sometimes seemed like a shadow version of herself. My sister and I worried that ALS was killing her, too.

We'd talk to my dad about bringing in even more help, and he'd balk and say, "Why? Mom is doing fine," and I'd say, "How is Mom doing fine?" and he'd say, "She went to Target just last week, she's getting out of the house." I don't blame him for this myopic viewpoint anymore, but I did at the time. I think I said something like, "She went to fucking Target?—is that the sign of a rich and fulfilling life?"

He was literally trapped inside his body, so we understood the challenge he faced: all he wanted was one working finger, just one, so he could scroll through his fantasy baseball team's results, but instead he was forced to call for my mom, or me, or Ryan, to scroll for him. The disease didn't cause this blindness in my dad; it intensified it. He'd always been someone who had a plan for how he wanted to spend his time, but he didn't consult anyone else; we were just sort of expected to get on board. And he didn't like to be the butt of people's jokes or observations. In fact, whoever first uttered the phrase "You can dish it out, but you can't take it" was probably saying it to someone very much like my dad.

His fallibility doesn't seem all that important to me now. But it is important to share, as I know it would be to him. He was real, he could be difficult, he sometimes made people feel shitty but more often he made them feel important and amazing. And for each moment he wallowed in bitterness and anger about ALS, there were a dozen in which he did something that made me realize he possessed a humor and strength that I hope like hell to have at my end.

PART

Chapter 19

GOOD PEOPLE, BAD TIMES

*G*oing out for a ride had always been a pastime for my dad. When we were kids, he'd usually bribe us with a stop at an ice cream shop, sometimes one thirty or forty minutes away. He liked everything about these drives. He liked having his window down, fresh air and open roads, his left hand on the grab handle; he liked looking for birds out the window; he loved our company, and he'd reach his hand to the back seat and squeeze our toes. Then, as we got older and bigger, our calves.

We took these drives in the winter, too, but I only think of them in summer, in the same way some foreign countries seem, in the collective consciousness, to perpetually exist in one season—like Russia, which routinely evokes images of icy streets and fur coats. And so, for me, these rides are all freshly cut grass and the voice of Tim McCarver, the former play-by-play announcer for the New York Mets.

Going out for a ride in the mobility van was a hollow facsimile of what my dad once loved, and that fact wasn't lost on me each time we made the arduous journey from hospital bed to wheelchair to house ramp to driveway to van ramp to chair lock mechanism. Whatever sense of freedom the fresh air first offered my dad was exhausted by the time his neck, over which he now had almost no control, was sent bobbling as we thrust him into his passenger spot.

The van, which of course we never wanted, cost three times the price of any other car we'd bought. The company that sold us the van removed the front passenger seat and the middle row so we could, just barely, drive my dad's motorized wheelchair up the side ramp, spin him toward the front, and lock him into the open passenger space. My mom became adept at this maneuver, her eyes focused on each movement of the tiny joystick like it was a video game—an extremely challenging one. Every few days, my dad's foot would get pinned on a turn and he'd try to get our attention, though his voice was growing weaker. I would be watching as his ankle caught on the door at a gruesome angle, a replay in slow motion, and my mom would be trying to swivel him through, wrenching it more. My dad's eyes would be wide because he was completely at our mercy. In these moments, his fear became an energy. It wasn't isolated and focused, but deep and wide, and it would crash over us like a wave.

This panic bubbled to the surface each time we left the house, but especially around the van. He had to trust us to protect every inch of a body over which he had no control but through which he could still feel pain. Think how clumsy we are in handling each other with the big things, like our hearts; now imagine turning over every movement of your body to someone else.

It was while driving that my dad had always been most contemplative. And now that he was at the cliff's edge, I craved knowledge about the view and how it changed how he thought about life. He had never been a big "silver linings" guy. He bristled when people asked him tone-deaf questions such as, "What's your favorite part about being in a wheelchair?" (a real question), or when people ignorant of ALS suggested that a positive attitude and hard work would have him back on his feet in no time—this one particularly stinging because the disease was already devouring his sense of self, his belief that he was strong of mind and body.

But he did begin to cherish small pleasures that previously he might have only casually noticed. This seemingly minor difference, cherishing instead of noticing, upgraded the quality of his days, making them manageable. Feeling the sun on his skin, smelling freshly made coffee, hearing one of his favorite songs, the sensation of a hand on his—these became almost holy to him. He would close his eyes as if he'd never experienced anything so wonderful.

I've always thought the concept of "silver linings" was a tricky one. Sometimes the cloud that passes overhead isn't too dark, and the positive side effects can immediately be gleaned and appreciated. But other times the cost of life's unexpected turn is so steep, and the positive side effects so paltry, that the two can't be bridged. And then, at first, asking for silver linings feels almost offensive. The only thing that closes that chasm is time. When he was first diagnosed, my dad could not name a single positive side effect; by the end, he could name many. At the top of that list were the people surrounding him and the unexpected ways they loved and cared for him.

And on this day, in that cursed mobility van, my dad seemed more philosophical than usual. I was driving, my right hand across the console, resting on his forearm. He was without his oxygen mask for a few minutes, so I could more easily hear him.

"Through all this, I've realized one thing is true," he said.

Thirsty for insight, my eyes flew to his: "Oh yeah? What's that?"

"It's true what people say: You do find good people in bad times and bad people in good times. The people we've found during this time, specifically Mary Rose and Jeanine, they are so good, and they are so good to me, and I appreciate them so much. They are good people in a bad time, and good people show up in bad times—I've found this to be very true."

I thought of my own life, of the agents who started calling once I began doing TV at ESPN, eager to profit, but who stopped calling once I left ESPN. The friends who showed up, day in and day out, regardless of what job I held or how much money I made, but then also the people I thought were friends who dropped me once I couldn't do much for them anymore. Perhaps I had been that opportunistic person in someone else's life, and I vowed never to be that person again.

Jeanine, my dad's nighttime aide, walked into our house every night at 7 p.m. She would place her phone and keys by the door, then turn excitedly toward my dad, like she couldn't wait to see him— this even though she'd already worked a full day and hadn't yet been home to see her kids. My dad would take her in, his eyes lifted upward like he was at a drive-in movie, as she told him the story of her day or the funny thing her daughters had done the night before. The first night they met, my dad told her how much he loved the TV show *Peaky Blinders,* and the next night Jeanine walked in saying, "Chris, oh my god, the Shelby family—you don't wanna cross them!" Delighted she had watched the show, my dad grinned and asked what episode she was on, and their rapport only grew from there.

You find good people in bad times and bad people in good times.

I thought of Mary Rose, his daytime aide, who was never a minute late in the mornings, the person my dad trusted more than anyone to keep him safe when using the machine that lifted him from bed to wheelchair. Soft-spoken and gentle, she giggled at all of my dad's jokes, which he delivered in the hope of breaking through her natural shyness. Most mornings as Mary Rose got ready to move him, he'd call out to Google Assistant: "Hey, Google, play 'Growin' Up' by Bruce Springsteen." The song would begin playing, and Mary Rose would roll my dad gently onto his side so she could slide the harness beneath him. Once the contraption was in place, she'd maneuver the lever and he'd be airlifted, suspended between bed and wheelchair for a few seconds. He had decided this considerable operation needed its own soundtrack.

At the end of the live version of "Growin' Up," Springsteen speaks to the crowd, yelling, "It was bye-bye, New Jersey, we were airborne!" He stretches out the last word: *aiiiiirbooorne*. My dad's goal was to synchronize Springsteen's lyrics with his transfer. I can still hear him calling from the living room, "And The Big C is airborne!" and Mary Rose giggling softly by his side.

You find good people in bad times and bad people in good times.

RITUAL AND ROUTINE

*I*n my body there's a poem taught to me by my dad, though I per-fected it myself. Such a poem exists inside every basketball player, a series of movements executed each time they step to the free throw line.

I walk to the line. I hold the ball on my left hip as I set my right foot on the small mark that represents the line's, and therefore the rim's, precise center. I do not yet look up at the hoop. I spin the ball in my hands, then turn until I see the label—Spalding or Nike or Wilson—and place my right hand across the graphic. I bend my knees and quickly dribble twice. I pause, and then, and only then, do I finally look at the rim, after I am already in motion upward.

I will never forget this sequence of movements, the flow of them, how right they feel to me, my dad's guidance at each stage.

This wasn't the only routine, or ritual, introduced by my dad; it's just the only one I can physically express. In that way it feels distinctive, as if each time I perform this choreography I prove his existence. (How else would I know these movements, universe?)

Everything else plays on a screen in my mind. Some moments exist in my memory for reasons I don't understand. A late-summer walk, for example, that I took alone to the dark blue mailbox around the corner from my house, a flimsy letter in hand. What was it about that afternoon, I wonder, that my brain felt compelled to save? Were the colors bolder, the leaves in peak pigment, the earthy smell of freshly cut grass richer? There are a million moments I'd rather remember than this. And yet when I examine it further a feeling arises: the long stretch of those empty summer days; the growing grass and heat and mosquito bites; and me, a kid, floating along on a dense fog of pre-technology boredom that now feels mysterious and inaccessible.

So then, maybe this moment does matter. Maybe it's my access point into a much larger file: middle school summers. If that is true, my file "Life with Dad" has numerous access points. Sometimes it feels like he read a handbook, How to Make a Kid Reminisce about Childhood, *because my recollections aren't one-offs, they are layered, a thousand similar memories laid on top of one another until the result becomes something like 3D. And then I close my eyes and press Play.*

My dad is rolling down his window before putting the car in reverse. Both of us are drenched in sweat. I buckle my seat belt, toss the ball into the back seat. Without even looking at him, I know he's smiling. The aura of his smile fills the car. Nothing could spoil his good mood after playing basketball, and nothing was better than Dad in a good mood.

I hold my hand out the window, try to catch the breeze. We approach the corner convenience shop, Stewart's, with its deep brown brick exterior, its handwritten advertisements for gallons of milk and dozens of eggs. He flips the blinker for a left turn and slides the car into the front parking spot.

"I buy, you fly?" he says, even though I know this ritual by heart, even though words aren't necessary. He says them because not saying

them is like forgetting to attach the key words to a search result—the memory might be filed wrong, and we can't have that. We are building something here, after all.

I am young and he is less young, so I dart inside with two dollars in my hand and a deep, basketball-induced thirst that needs quenching. Do I love basketball, or do I love standing in front of a wall of ice-cold Gatorade? I don't know. But in my mind, it all becomes one: Dad, basketball, sweat, open windows, I-buy-you-fly, Gatorade.

This moment happened a thousand times. I open the case and grab an orange, a lemon-lime, a fruit punch, a Glacier Freeze, a Riptide Rush. Then the feeling of slipping back into the car, handing Dad his drink, twisting the top off mine—ahhhhhhh.

My dad rendered it layer upon layer upon layer, so that now I access it in Technicolor.

Chapter 20

MORPHINE

At the end of April my dad had a feeding tube inserted. This was his second hospitalization, after being rushed to the emergency room with the blood clot in January. More hospital trips would be coming. The muscles controlling his swallowing mechanism had been weakening for months, to the point where each bite felt risky. He was choking frequently. This procedure was the first lifesaving intervention my dad chose. At this mile marker, some ALS patients decide against any invasive measures, call in hospice, and slowly fade away. But my dad believed that if he could grin and bear it long enough, maybe a cure would come rushing down the pipeline. He didn't want to be the guy who sold the stock just before it rocketed upward. He was trying to balance preparing for death and fighting for life, though I wondered if these two things might genuinely be mutually exclusive.

After the surgery my dad was allowed morphine every four hours. He wasn't sure he needed the drug for pain relief, as it was intended, and neither was I. But we did know that after the first dose, he fell asleep for two consecutive hours—the longest stretch of uninterrupted sleep in months. Surely, insomnia is also a form of pain.

I was staying overnight in the hospital to relieve my mom, who needed a full night's sleep at home. Our family was extremely protective of our dad, and we likely wouldn't have left him alone overnight regardless of the disease, but ALS presented particular challenges in that he couldn't move his arms and therefore couldn't hit the call button, and his voice was too weak to carry to the hallway.

Among my jobs on the overnight shift was to find the nurse every three hours and forty-five minutes to remind her of the upcoming morphine dose. The clock was directly in my dad's sightline, and he was stalking the minute hand. This rapid shift into addictive behavior surprised me—I'd never seen him take anything stronger than Advil—but I didn't begrudge him. Honestly, I was shocked it had taken that long for him to upgrade to an opioid. Anything that gave him a moment of relief, I'd advocate for.

I found the nurse, and she wheeled her mobile computer station into my dad's room and hovered over his bed.

"What number would you say the pain is?" she asked.

I could see a moment of hesitation while he calculated what number would get him the morphine without setting off alarm bells and, equally important, without sacrificing the pride he felt as an athlete with high pain tolerance. Telling her that the pain was a 10 was not an option.

"A seven," he said, and he knew he'd gambled a little bit. Was 7 high enough to warrant the morphine? He wasn't sure. But he hoped he'd hit the sweet spot: sense of self shaken—since when is he someone who dissembles to get morphine?—but not shattered.

The nurse typed something into her computer, then promised to be back at the top of the hour with the dose. After she left, he let out a breath and stared at the ceiling.

"Hey," I said, putting my hand on his. "I love you." I'd discovered there were plenty of wrong things to say, but I love you was never one of them.

"This is just—wow," he said. "I keep thinking about how mom and I would go see her dad when he was in a nursing home. We'd be there trying to visit with him, but it seemed like all he cared about was watching the clock for when he could get his next dose of morphine. God, I was so judgmental of him—the lack of willpower, the dependency on a substance. It felt like a character flaw. It felt like weakness. I was disgusted by it. And now I'm—" he turned his eyes to mine; he was still swimming back from the memory.

"—I'm staring at the clock, just like he once did. Why did I think I had the right to judge him? How could I have thought I knew what he was going through?"

I waited for him to say something more, but he was deep in his own mind. His eyes went back to the ceiling. He was churning through the memory, over and over, processing the ramifications on his belief system. He was wondering how he had made this mistake, how he could have gotten something so obvious so wrong.

Chapter 21

NO SURRENDER

My fixation on the concept of surrender began with a phone call to a friend, Dana Childs, who also works as an empath—she connects to a deep source and reads people's spirit and energy. I'd scheduled time for us to talk because I was spiraling about my dad's disease. It just made no sense. The cruelty of it left me confused: Why would ALS exist at all?

In college I'd flirted with born-again Christianity—it was all the rage among my basketball teammates—but since then, I'd been decidedly agnostic. Then I met Kathryn. She encouraged me to consider something bigger than just evolutionary randomness, than just—*bam!*—lights out. And of course, since one of my favorite people was at death's door, I became more open to concepts of a higher power, in which I desperately wanted to believe.

One such idea was reincarnation, which included ideas of source, spirit, and energy. Not many Buddhist principles have penetrated the American sports landscape, which is perhaps why even writing those words, *source* and *spirit,* causes me to flinch. In the world of athletics, the higher powers are Jesus Christ and hard work, and not necessarily in that order.

The connective tissue, the single character trait, that links great athletes is luck. As in, almost none of them believe it exists. Think about it. Most of us understand how luck informs our lives, but most of the best athletes in the world won't even touch that logic. I can stand here and believe that a world exists in which Kobe Bryant is drafted No. 13 to the Charlotte Hornets, isn't traded to the Lakers, gets stuck on a bad team, maybe gets an injury, and he's out of the league in five, six years. But in Bryant's mind, on every planet in the multiverse, he molded himself into an eighteen-time All-Star with five NBA championships.

You can't be one of the greatest of all time, standing there with the ball, seven seconds left, and allow yourself to believe that luck will have anything to do with what happens next. Surrendering to the whims of fate, or the lesson the universe is teaching you, is in many ways antithetical to the ethos of an athlete, who fosters an inner strength and resiliency regardless of circumstance. And there's that word again: *surrender.* It keeps company with *weakness* and *quitting* and *losing,* all seen as moral failings in the sports world and beyond. Here was the delicate paradox: I became obsessed with surrender when my perception of it was turned on its head. I started viewing giving in (or setting aside the fight or no longer fighting) as the greatest sign of strength.

Dana introduced me to the idea. I am naturally rational, and somewhat cynical, looking to poke holes in other people's concepts and beliefs. But seeing my dad's disease in action delivered a dose of humility. ALS just did not give a fuck about work ethic and perseverance.

After having the feeding tube inserted and recovering with the help of morphine, my dad was transferred to a rehabilitation facility where he—and where all of us—would learn how to manage his new reality. Before this surgery, which was in early April, he could still walk—to the car and back, no more, just enough to keep some semblance of quality of life. But after nearly ten days in the hospital, which included a staph infection, he couldn't stand without the help of two people. Because he was an athlete, he believed in rehab; that with the right mindset, he could regain his strength.

The night before being transferred to rehab, he looked me in the eyes as if swearing a solemn oath, and he said, "Katie, I promise you, I'm going to give it everything I have. I'm going to work as hard as I ever have." He looked so much like a little kid, begging for another chance, trying to convince me he was worthy. To prove his point he tried flexing the working muscle in his right arm and said, "Feel that muscle," and of course I smiled, remembering the thousands of times I'd been prompted over the years to confirm his strength.

An hour later, as I walked through the airport to my gate, I had to pause and lean against a railing, my eyesight blurry with tears. What crushed me was the earnestness, and futility, of his hope. Hard work solves most problems. But it could not solve this one.

I shared this story with Dana, and I told her my mind and heart were open. My earthbound belief structure of show-me-a-peer-reviewed-paper was currently failing me. I possessed no judgment about the concepts of higher spirit, energy, source, reincarnation—I just wanted to learn, from her perspective, why this was happening and how I could help my dad. We talked for a few minutes, and I explained that one of my most difficult challenges was the utter lack of hope. All my dad wanted was a sliver of a chance. Just a little daylight between disease and outcome. Was that too much to ask?

"What I'm hearing, what your dad's spirit is telling me, is that the lesson he came here to learn is surrender," Dana said. "I'm sensing that your dad is incredibly stubborn and hardworking, and teaching him the lesson of surrender was never going to be easy. Perhaps this was the only disease through which he stood a chance of learning. Often, the life we're given seems counterintuitive to the lesson we're meant to learn. For example, if your spirit wanted you to learn about freedom, you might assume you'd live an open life without restraint, on the road maybe, basking in the sun. But very often, the only way to learn the true value of freedom is to spend a life without it. It's only then, when you're allowed to taste true freedom after captivity, that you can really understand what it means."

Until right then, I believed that on the other side of surrender (or losing, or failing, or quitting) existed a weakened version of yourself. But what if, Dana was encouraging me to consider, the act of surrendering (or losing, or failing, or quitting) was a show of strength. What if it actually brought you closer to your true self?

Dana spoke the word *surrender* as if it was sacred. She was not using it as some kind of get-out-of-jail-free card. A hard-won truth is what it sounded like on her lips, in the same family as perseverance and freedom and compassion and generosity.

I realized the damage done when messaging from the outside world trumps your inner voice. I'd long ago decided to agree with what the outside world told me: giving up, quitting, walking away, surrendering, these were evidence of weakness, and, should I choose them, I would find a lesser version of myself.

How long I had labored over my decision to leave ESPN despite knowing, for more than a year, that I must go. But I needed time, I told myself, to brace for the lesser version of me on the other side. I would become someone who hit Pause on their life, who didn't have a plan. No matter the people around me who insisted the decision would take strength; my social conditioning ran deep. *Surrendering to the unknown,* I believed, was some bullshit that people said because they didn't have the discipline to control their lives. I was not someone who surrendered—to the unknown, or to anything. And neither was my dad. But suddenly I was seeing it completely differently. Surrender, I'd decided, translated to peace. It was a peaceful show of strength. I wanted my dad to see it this way, and my attempts at making this so became increasingly comical.

For the last stretch of his life, when I was with him every other week, we'd drive to our lake house once a visit. My parents had bought the property—the first splurge of their lives—about five years earlier. They were so proud of the house: evidence of their dedication to each other and to the life they hoped to keep living. He loved the house, nestled deep in the trees. And so even once he could no longer walk, we would still push him out to the deck so he could look at the view of Lake George.

On the drive up we'd often listen to the Springsteen Channel on SiriusXM radio. The Boss holds a special place in my parents' hearts, as he had performed at Colgate University in 1976, back before he became a megastar and back when they were all just kids. One of Springsteen's most popular songs is titled "No Surrender," and it plays frequently on his channel because it never went radio mainstream—it's the ultimate insider's track. The song is beautiful, with astute lyrics. But at that moment in my life, the track's refrain felt like enemy propaganda. Springsteen sings:

> We made a promise, we swore we'd always remember
> No retreat, baby, no surrender
> Like soldiers in the winter's night with a vow to defend
> No retreat, baby, no surrender.

I'm sure that earlier in life I'd have considered this my anthem. But on those drives, I'd see the song title pop onto the dashboard screen,

I'd recognize the opening chords, and I'd let out a long sigh. Then I'd glance next to me, at my dad trapped in his chair, and notice that he'd already registered what was playing.

The first time we heard it together, I changed the channel after the first minute. I tried to act like the decision was unplanned, like I was just looking for something better. My dad immediately balked and asked me to put it back on, and of course I did. As soon as the song ended, he explained that it was now *his anthem*. "It reminds me that I have to stay tough, that I can't let this disease beat me," he said. "No defeat, baby, no surrender."

On other days, sitting on the couch next to his hospital bed, I'd actually say, "What do you think about just...surrendering?" I'd say this as if it had just popped into my mind and I was trying it on for size. *We could try, I don't know...surrendering?* It's not a casual idea, but I tried to make it so. Each time, my dad would look confused. "I've lived my life one way, Katie, and that's never giving up," he would say. "How could I possibly, at the very end, throw in the towel? This part of who I am, it's one of the last pieces of me left."

But what if, I wondered, what if surrendering isn't the giving up of everything that came before, but rather the *gathering up*?

At some point it dawned on me: the kind of surrendering I'd discovered, and that my dad would also eventually discover, comes from the inside out, not the other way around.

Chapter 22

THE PERFORMANCE

One night, while back home in Charleston, I decided to make tea. After pouring hot water into the mug, I was returning the electric kettle to its holder when, somehow, it slipped out of my hand and landed on my favorite item in the kitchen: an old dish in the shape of Corsica—a gift from my dad.

The plate broke into three pieces.

The only accurate way to describe what happened next—and who cares if it's a cliché—is to say that I burst into tears. My wife was sitting on the couch just a few yards away. She popped up.

"Was that the Corsica plate?" she asked, already halfway to the kitchen.

I nodded dramatically. I remember this weird feeling taking over, as if I was *performing* sadness as much as I was actually sad. And in the next second, I remember wondering how common this feeling was—how much energy grieving people spend wondering how their grief is being interpreted by others. Wondering if they're "doing it right," if it's justified. Of course, my goal after the plate broke wasn't to *be dramatic;* my body was just suddenly incapable of subtle movement. My eyes became big and wet; my head dropped; my shoulders sagged.

The plate had been broken for only a few seconds, but already I'd accepted and rejected the symbolism of its breaking multiple times. *(No, the plate does not represent my dad. Well, it kind of feels like it does. A plate is not a person. But things do have energy . . .)*

Eventually I wore myself down and accepted the symbolism—I let the breaking of the plate break me. And there, next to me, appeared my wife to piece me back together. She wrapped me in a hug.

"I'll fix it," she said.

"You can't fix it," I said.

"We'll get superglue tomorrow and I'll fix it," she said. "You'll see."

Unsaid between us: *But that's not really what's broken.*

(She knew that, of course. But we must fix what we can—because we can. And so she fixed it. And now our Corsica plate is functional again, with seams of glue, and back in its original spot, to the left of the stove.)

This wasn't the only time I found myself seemingly trapped between staged play and reality. Six months later I held my dad's foot in my hands and gently lowered it into the warm water. The door to his ICU room was closed and the curtain next to his bed was pulled shut; it was just the two of us. I was sitting at the base of his hospital bed, and I began washing his toes with a hand towel. He closed his eyes and I imagined—I hoped—that the heat of the water, that my hands on his skin, was calming him.

But I was also watching myself wash him. I tried not to let it happen, tried to stay present, but I couldn't help feeling like I was acting out a scene in some movie script: long-lost daughter (not quite) cleans feet of dying (was he?) father. I tried telling myself I possessed no ulterior motive—it was just a simple kindness, no big deal; his feet needed cleaning, and here I was. But my mind kept churning through all the layers of self-awareness, wondering how much I was motivated by love and service, how much by the desire to create and briefly live inside an intimate moment that told the story of *devoted daughter.* Honestly, I couldn't have said.

I tried turning off this debilitating metaview. *Not everything needs deconstructing,* I chided myself. But as I was washing my dad's feet, I could never shake the feeling that I was both reacting to life and artificially constructing a scene at the same time. As I dried one foot, then lifted it back to the bed, I wondered if this was just how the mind processes deeply emotional moments: by initially duping us into feeling that we've parachuted onto the stage in an alternate universe.

Of course I wasn't washing the feet of my dad, who was trapped inside an immobile body, tethered to a breathing machine, dying of amyotrophic lateral sclerosis—that would just be ludicrous, that would be some glitch in the matrix, a quick glimpse meant to knock some perspective into me before order was restored. (But in the meantime, just in case, I would play my part with vigor.) In the real version of my life, my dad was still teaching me how to play basketball, still taking me out for ice cream cones, for dinner, still calling me three times a day, still waiting for me to come help him mow the yard.

I emptied the basin into the room's tiny silver sink, refilled it with fresh warm water, and carefully lowered his other foot into it. He didn't open his eyes, but I thought I heard him sigh peacefully. Obviously, deep down, I knew the moment was real. And it was precisely because I knew it was real that my mind was constructing barriers between me and its emotional impact. My brain just didn't want to sit still in that reality.

Later he told me the moment between us had felt "biblical," and he looked at me softly, and that made me feel both warm and fuzzy and exposed, because I'd secretly hoped he'd been moved by the gesture. Questioning my motivations became routine: How much of what I was doing was for me, so I could feel like, and be seen as, a good kid, and how much was solely for him? I could never precisely tell the difference—still can't. But now I realize that it doesn't matter; it's all part of the trick the mind plays—the glitch in the system—that tries to insulate, and distract, from the rawness of death.

When we were kids, my sister and I were playing indoors with a Nerf football when we inadvertently knocked over an item of my dad's: a porcelain doll wearing a Colgate University basketball uniform. The doll landed on its head and broke into a hundred pieces. Worried we had ruined something important to him, the two of us spent the rest of the day rebuilding the doll's head, piecing it together with Elmer's glue. When we finished, the head still had a few missing pieces. The doll looked like something out of a horror movie, but my dad kept it. Not because he had ever really liked it (he hadn't), but because he was so charmed by our teamwork and perseverance.

What motivated us that long-ago day? Love of our dad, certainly. But also fear of his anger and disappointment, and distress over being viewed as irresponsible. Most pronounced in my memory, though, was the childlike belief that if we tried hard enough, we could make the doll look brand-new. And on some deep level, I don't think I ever stopped believing that.

Chapter 23

BE WITH MY PEOPLE

I flipped to the last page of my notebook, uncapped my pen, and began writing. "Dear Dad," I wrote, then paused. I was ashamed about what I needed to write, stunned that I'd penned a letter expressing that, maybe, possibly, my dad should choose to die. I outlined the reasons I was against my dad getting a tracheostomy—a surgery that would take his voice, attach him to a ventilator, and necessitate 24-7 care. He was scheduled for this operation in just a few days.

A month earlier we had presented him with two options. We could call in hospice, keep him at home, and make him comfortable for however long he had left. Or, he could have this surgery and extend his life—possibly for years. This second option came with the abovementioned caveats (no voice, around-the-clock care), as well as an additional one: the ALS would keep progressing anyway.

"I feel like I'm in a nightmare," he had said. "How can I choose between these two options? These aren't even options. There must be another way."

And, for a while, there was: doing nothing. What he "wanted" was to perfectly time the surgery so he could wring out as much quality of life as possible. Essentially, he was playing a game of chicken, and every passing day we were that much closer—how close, we couldn't know—to the oncoming train.

But the muscles that pumped air in and out of his lungs continued to weaken, and now he could rarely spend more than a few minutes without his breathing mask. He'd already told us that he wanted to be kept alive by all measures, so over several conversations we convinced him: if the outcome, either way, meant he would be put on a ventilator, scheduling the surgery proactively gave us more control of the variables.

He finally agreed, and my mom booked the surgery for the following week. Even though we'd presented the tracheostomy as a viable option, now that it was my dad's chosen course, I was surprised by how blindsided I felt. *Is this really happening?* I wondered. Suddenly, the train was barreling down the track.

The four of us—my mom, my dad, Ryan, and me—were gathering that night for a family meeting, another oddity introduced by ALS. We had never been a "family meeting" kind of family. I was terrified of the ventilator, and I needed to say so. My main concern was the fatigue and fear that was already drowning all of us. Just the night before, my mom and I went for a walk, trying to reconcile what life would look like on the other side of the surgery. The hospital bed and ventilator forever in the living room, someone by my dad's bed every minute, my parents' life savings dwindling, my dad trapped inside a body that couldn't move or talk and my mom tethered to his bedside.

"This is his decision," my mom kept saying. "It's his life. Nobody can make the decision for him."

"But Mom," I said. "This can't be the rest of our lives—this can't be the rest of *your* life."

"I'm okay, Kate," she said. "I'm ready for it. Whatever he decides now, that's not your burden to carry; it's mine. You need to go back to living your life."

I stopped walking. We were on a suburban street corner, no one in sight. My mom turned to check on me as I brought my hands to my face and screamed into them. The sound seemed to bounce around the neighborhood. My mom didn't even appear surprised by my outburst. She just gently placed a hand on my back and a couple seconds later we kept walking.

The first time I remember going for a run, I was with my dad. We did a loop of about two miles, but as we were jogging the straight-away toward our driveway, my dad looked at his watch and saw that the time was 19:37. Nineteen minutes, thirty-seven seconds.

"Gotta keep running," he said. "We'll go past the house until we hit twenty minutes, nice and even." I didn't balk at this logic. Of course we would run an extra few yards so we could hit a round number. And once we did, I made my dad show me his watch so I could feel the satisfaction of seeing the number. He was right: running 20:00 felt so much better than running 19:37. As if the difference wasn't just a few seconds, but actually everything—between a good run and not running at all. This was how things were done in our family: we didn't just run through the finish line; we sometimes ran past it. Picture me, at every year of my life, running a few yards past my stopping point just so I could hit that blissful round number, endorphins seemingly trapped behind those triple zeros like a slot machine jackpot.

Maybe this helps explain my reaction on that walk with my mom. I felt conquered. When it came to my dad, I wanted to run the full course with him. Hell, I even wanted to run that extra bit. But a ventilator? That would extend the course another ten miles, and if he did that, I would have to stop running, look down at my watch, and see a fractured number. If that happened, it would feel like I hadn't shown up for him at all.

I was angry at him for this. That's not fair, and I know it makes me seem selfish, but honestly, I was angry. Instead of being the daughter who played her heart out until the end, I would become the daughter who gave up, who didn't have the stamina. He was going to steal something from me. For the past year I'd been playing the game as if just a few minutes were left on the clock. I know that to some extent my sister and mom felt the same way. I was on an airplane, on average, every three days, and my marriage was mostly on pause. When I was with my dad, I slept on the couch next to him, getting only a few hours of rest a night. And when I wasn't there, my mom slept (or didn't sleep) in the same spot. My sister had moved her family from Boston, was working remotely, and was trying to raise two kids.

The only saving grace was the knowledge that it couldn't go on much longer. But then came the concept of the tracheostomy, and suddenly no finish line existed. To restore the quality of our lives, my dad's needed to end—the last, cruel mindfuck of a disease filled with mindfucks. My mom, my sister, and I talked endlessly about the decision before us—before him, really—and I hated myself for believing only one reasonable decision existed.

My sister and I would often meet at Starbucks and talk. And on this day, with my red notebook opened to its final page, she pushed through the front door, and upon spotting her, I quickly closed the cover. She sat next to me, and we proceeded to have a version of a conversation we'd had dozens of times before. Except this time, she articulated something I had never managed to name.

I had been thinking about our situation in terms of numbers, which Ryan also appreciated: "Essentially," I said, "if Dad goes through with the tracheostomy, his quality of life's gonna go down from something like four percent to one percent—barely any quality of life at all. And in order to keep him at that one percent quality of life, it's going to cost mom ninety percent of her quality of life and, say, fifty percent each of *our* quality of life. So that's—what?"—I quickly added ninety and fifty and fifty—"one hundred ninety percentage points of quality of life, all to keep Dad hovering at one percentage point."

"I know, I know," she said, then looked away. When she looked back, she added: "But for him, that one percentage point is…every-thing."

Oh, she was right. How much collective quality of life was our family willing to spend to keep my dad's single percentage point? No equation could solve that problem.

That night, the three of us gathered around my dad's wheelchair. Open on my lap was my red notebook. As he did at the beginning of all these meetings, my dad took on the affect of a man under ambush—partly for comedic effect, partly because that's how he felt. "Oh, no," he'd say. "This must be bad if the Three Amigos want to see me."

Of course, he was a captive audience. I looked at the letter I'd written. My mom and Ryan knew its contents, and while they agreed with the sentiment in principle, they were less sure of its need to be spoken. In particular, my mom had told me she couldn't bear personally saying anything that might make him feel she (or we) didn't adore him enough to take on this burden. But I still felt I needed to say something.

I was sitting in a kitchen chair in front of my dad, my mom had her arm across my dad's shoulder and was attempting to lean against his chair, and my sister was on the corner of the couch. We formed a tight circle. Although earlier, in Starbucks, I'd been able to transcribe my concerns, now I wasn't sure I'd be able to speak them aloud. So, we started easy.

"We just wanted to talk about the decision to move forward with the tracheostomy," I said. Dad nodded. His nose and mouth were covered by his breathing mask. "We just want to make sure we talk openly about the impact of this decision, first and foremost on you, but also on us as a family. Make sure everything is out on the table."

This seemed to scare him—you could see it in his eyes—and he tried to speak through the mask: "We've...already...talked...and...decided?" His voice was so weak he needed to pause between words.

For the next ten minutes we danced around the hot core of what needed to be said, trying not to get burned. Most of the thoughts I'd outlined in my letter were mentioned: the toll on Mom (at this, my dad looked softly at her), the sky-high monetary cost (was there a cost ceiling on his life?), the need for him to find purpose beyond just hoping for a cure (but *why?*, his eyes seemed to ask).

His world had become so small. It was hard to know how much of the bigger picture he was able to see.

Eventually the conversation started to come to its natural conclusion. Only I hadn't yet said what I needed to say. In my mind I considered Ryan's earlier comment about the incalculable value of Dad's final one percent. Maybe I didn't need to say anything at all; maybe what I wanted to say would only serve me; maybe I'd regret it for the rest of my life; maybe I'd regret not saying it.

"Wait," I interjected. "I have to say one more thing." I scooted my chair a few inches closer to my dad so I could place my hand on his knee. I looked at him and heard him say—his voice muffled beneath his mask—"Uh-oh."

"No matter what you decide, I will support you, and I will be there for you, and I will give everything I have to make it work. But I just need you to know that I—I don't want you to go on a ventilator. I'm scared for you, that you'll be trapped in a way you can't even imagine, and I'm scared for myself, and I'm scared for all of us—for what it will mean about the rest of our lives. I don't want you to do it, Dad. That's all."

I was looking right at him. And his eyes began filling. He started pressing his right foot, repeatedly, into the footrest of his chair, and my mom leaned down so she could hear him better. "You want the mask off?" she asked, and he nodded. A second later, she lifted it from his face, and I could now fully see the tears streaming down his cheeks.

"I don't…want…to leave…my people," he said, taking a moment to look at each of us. "I'm not…ready. I want…to be…around…my people."

We were his people. I was his people. And if one of my people needed me, I decided in that moment, then nothing else mattered. Not the time or the sleep or the money or my fear or my need for rounded, satisfying numbers and fully executed races and daughter-of-the-year awards.

"Then that's settled," we all said, laughing through tears. I walked into the kitchen and carefully tore out the last page of my notebook, ripped it into pieces, and put the torn paper into the trash.

Turns out, though, that placing words in the trash doesn't erase them from your memory. For the next day I walked around with a tightness in my chest. Had I been courageous, or had I been selfish? Was I a speaker of bold truths, or reckless with my words? I couldn't decide. I truly couldn't.

Then, a few hours before we had to leave for the hospital, a WhatsApp notification lit up my phone. I was downstairs in the basement, my dad above me on his eye gaze computer—this cool piece of technology that allowed him to type messages by following the movement of his eyes. Eagerly, I read his words:

> **Dad:** I totally understand your thoughts yesterday I don't want you to think that I think you love me less. I just am not ready for hospice I want to see how this will work

out for me I am going to take a deep breath tomorrow morning just like before a big shot.

Me: That made me cry. Thank you for sending me this. I love you so much and I am ready to support you, like down in a defensive crouch ready to go. (Not a low crouch because I don't totally love playing defense.)

Him: I'd feel a lot better if instead of playing defense for me, you were ready to take a big shot for me.

(I was a much better shooter than defender.)

Me: Thank you for this note, though. You made me feel so much better.

Him: I frequently think of our conversation on your wedding day. I would never stay mad.

Me: And I would never stay mad at you. Cause you're wonderful.

Him: And you've passed me the ball too many times.

Me: I have assisted on more baskets than anyone, I believe.

I read this exchange, and smile, at least once a week. As for that torn piece of paper, I've forgotten exactly what I wrote on it.

Chapter 24

THE UNPAID TRILLIONS

T he vision I had of caretakers, when I thought of caregiving at all, was something like this: a peaceful setting and an adoring woman—almost always a woman—tenderly spooning soup into a loved one's mouth. What I did not think of, what is rarely shown, is the solitude and sadness and resentment, the sleepless nights leading to zombie days, the endless administrative work, the pressure and fatigue, the loosening grip on reality. What I did not realize is that caregiving will swallow you whole, and that caretaking can kill you, unless another person steps in, charged with caring for the caretaker. (And even then...good luck.)

This is to say: I started worrying for my mom's life. My dad was dying, yes, but somewhere along the way I noticed that my mom was tethered to him, and that he believed he needed her there—for comfort, for ease, for love.

It's simple for me to remember a childhood spent in the gym with my dad, but only because my mom made that possible. Not that I noticed. The inner workings of our household, and who did what, happened mostly out of my sight. My dad was good at being the hero, and my mom was good at letting him. I realized this only after he got sick. My mom and I have always been close, but in a different way, because we are similar in the ways my dad and I are not: we love a philosophical discussion, an adventure, and spontaneity and impulsiveness. In fact, that last word, *impulsive,* if you go to its Latin root, means "driven onward," and nothing summarizes my mom and me better than that. We are always driven onward—to the next stop, the next event, the next thought, the next idea, the next moment.

Which is why seeing her tethered and stationary awakened something inside me. The truth, I realized only then, was that my dad had defined much of the first half of my life. Basketball, college, sports journalism, ESPN—all of these were a by-product of a childhood spent following him, absorbing his passions. But my mom? She shaped the passions instilled in us by him. My dad was a larger-than-life presence. But as he became increasingly sick, I started craving my mom. I had these visions of us traveling the world, long conversations over wine, digging into politics and spirituality, expanding each other's mind and perspective. It was clear to me: in the next chapter of life, I needed her.

I did not want my mom to go down with the ship. I don't think my dad did, either, but his perspective had dwindled to a keyhole, through which he only ever wanted to see my mom—giving him pills, fixing his pillows, helping clean him. But caregiving, I realized, was a zero-sum game: the only way to give my mom freedom was to sacrifice his comfort. Yet during that time, her freedom felt like a luxury, his comfort a necessity. (Maybe it had always been that way.)

Few people talk about the sticky dynamics of caregiving or of women's unpaid labor. (And FYI: studies value women's annual unpaid labor at $10.9 trillion worldwide, $1.5 trillion domestically.)

My sister and I, we could not see the wisdom of losing our mother to the hopeless cause of not losing our father. But we were not in their marriage, and the decisions they made together were not ours to judge. We did anyway, of course, and tried to pry open the door to let in some light. It wasn't easy. What my mom could say to me ("I can't keep doing this, I'm losing myself") she could not say to him.

I am lucky, we are lucky—in so many ways. But the one I'm thinking of now is that my dad always had my mom, until the last second, comforting and soothing him. And that while I watched her do all of this for him, surrendering herself, I started to see my mom differently. I began to understand what she had sacrificed all along, raising us in my dad's hometown, away from her family, letting him decree the pastimes of our household. These choices cost her in ways I'd never known. Death is a pressure cooker: hard truths get boiled down.

Chapter 25

GUINNESS

My dad could make a game of anything. Going out to dinner as little kids, my mom, my sister and I would scoot into the booth, then eagerly turn our full attention to him, excited to hear what entertainment he'd thought up. His games were never elaborate. Once, at a diner, he pulled out three sugar packets, used his fork to mark one of them, then proceeded to mesmerize us with an impromptu version of the shell game. I remember those sugar packets more clearly than our Nintendo 64. No matter the circumstance, my dad immediately put kids into a state of rapture. They clung to him. Sometimes I'd watch, trying to detect the magic sauce. What was it, exactly? I noted that he rarely needed or used props, just imagination and his full attention.

I can't remember when I stopped being good at play, but I'm not the only one noticing the loss. Play, in all its various forms, seems to be a dwindling commodity. By the end of middle school years, kids are usually serious about a sport. And while they "play" that sport, that's not *play*—not in the cosmic sense of the word. They're often playing for a résumé's sake, or college application's sake, or achievement culture's sake.

I would watch my dad with my nephew Henry, each of them pretending to be a wild animal, and wonder what was broken in me. Perhaps my dad was also just going through the motions, but he always made a convincing hippo. I started to wonder whether our culture had broken me. I'd been told to find my passion, make it my job, and I'd "never have to work a day in my life." But that's not the whole truth. Passion rarely survives obligation. Somewhere along the way, I'd forgotten where work ended and play began—or vice versa. I started to believe that even my play needed to have an endgame, an element of productivity. Sometimes as I watched my dad and Henry the whole thing just felt like another hustle. If I joined them, was I doing it for Instagram? So other people thought I was a good aunt? To check some box as a well-rounded adult? I just couldn't—I wasn't able—to play for play's sake.

But my dad, he could play until the very end. Once, the two of us had to drive to Syracuse—three hours away—and when I climbed into the car, he said, "Okay, here's what we're going to do. I'm going to swing by Record Town, drop you off in front with a twenty-dollar bill, and you're going to get us whatever CD you want—your choice—and we'll listen to it the whole ride." Inside the store, I checked out all the major displays— Destiny's Child, Third Eye Blind, Shania Twain—but I wanted to find something we'd both like. Then, turning around, I saw a stack of CDs: *Al Green's Greatest Hits*. There was Al Green on the cover, shirtless, pointing at the camera, and for some reason I thought, *That's the one!* When I climbed into the car and presented him with my selection, my dad was charmed. Surprised, but charmed. (It was 1998. He must have thought I'd return with the Backstreet Boys or Ace of Base.) That day, and for years afterward, we listened to the CD on repeat. Anytime Al Green came on the radio, Dad would turn to me and smile, or phone me and turn up the dial. And dozens of times, at parties or out to dinner with friends, he'd tell the story: "So, I send her in with twenty bucks and what does she come back with?"

For the life of me, I cannot remember why we had to drive to Syracuse, but it was like my dad understood the potential banality of the day and just couldn't abide such dullness. Climbing into the car that morning was like sliding into the booth as a little kid, my eyes drawn to him, wondering what kind of fun he'd dreamed up for us.

So, I shouldn't have been surprised when he tried to put an entertaining twist on what he knew would be the worst day of his life. It was about a week before the surgery that would take away his voice, as well as his ability to eat and drink, and I walked in the door from the airport to see my mom huddled beside my dad's wheelchair. They looked like co-conspirators.

"What is it?" I put down my bag.

They looked at each other, then my mom said to me, "Dad has an idea."

"Tell Kate," my mom said to him, but he was stuck behind his oxygen mask and he said, between breaths, "You...tell...her."

"Your dad had the very cool idea of making a commercial. The night before he goes in for the trach, we're going to pour a glass of Guinness, then he's going to explain to the camera that he's decided that the last thing he ever wants to taste is...Guinness! It'll be like a viral video—you know, like if you had to decide the last thing you'd ever taste, what would it be?"

"That sounds amazing," I said, and he smiled and nodded behind his mask. I noticed that his plan had a few hurdles: his voice was almost gone, as was his ability to swallow. But those things mattered less than the energy behind the gesture. He was bringing his playful attitude to a dreadful circumstance.

The night before his surgery, we set up the scene. We poured out mugs of Guinness for all of us. My dad, using his eyes, typed his script into his text-to-voice machine. Then, when he was ready, we took off his breathing mask, hit Record, and his automated voice filled the air: "If you could choose one last food, one last drink, what might it be? Tonight, I face the choice and I choose a Guinness. Sláinte. Tomorrow, I face a tracheostomy." Then my mom brought the straw, suspended in his mug of beer, to his lips. He closed his eyes to marshal the strength to draw the Guinness into his mouth, and a moment later—as often happened after he swallowed something— he started coughing. I ended the recording a second later.

The production quality wasn't as high as I'd hoped. Plus, a commercial is less persuasive when its star coughs up the product at the end. The video is still on my phone, and I've never sent it to anyone— not even my mom or sister. For a long time, I'd scroll through my photos, see the square with that video, and pretend I hadn't. When I thought of it, I thought of my dad hoping, but failing, to make one last mark on the world. And did he know, as he choked on that sip of Guinness, that his idea had fallen flat?

Chris Fagan was an ordinary man dying in an extraordinary way, and I kept wondering if he really hoped the video would go viral so that even at the end he could spread the good word about who he was and the things he loved. Maybe I was the one bringing my global objectives to his homemade video. Maybe I was the one obsessed with scale, influence, and outside validation. All he'd ever worried about was making the things around him good, and on that night, maybe he sensed we needed that from him again: a little game to make a dreary day brighter, a flash of the old dad.

What never disappoints me is this: the memory of slipping into a booth with my mom and sister, blissed out over a fork-poked sugar packet, enthralled by my dad's imagination and undivided attention, the world beautifully ordinary.

That's the equation, I tell myself, then desperately try not to forget.

Lesson #8

LET ME BE YOUR FLUNKY

*E*very summer I would play in weekend-long AAU basketball tournaments. Picture a field house with three or more courts, each of them filled with young girls, their parents and siblings packing the sidelines and baselines. Between games we'd go to lunch or walk to the parking lot, where someone's van was filled with snacks and sports drinks. This was the late '90s, and everyone carried black Nike drawstring backpacks, inside which we'd put our sneakers and an extra T-shirt. I had a dozen teammates, and they all walked around wearing their little backpacks. But I almost never did. My dad wouldn't let me.

After a game I'd walk over to the bleachers or sideline where I'd left my stuff, and he'd meet me there. At this time, he was probably about forty years old and still one of the best players in the area. I'd put on a clean T-shirt and stuff my sneakers into my bag, then sling it over my shoulder.

"Let me get that," he'd say, holding out his hand.

"No, that's okay," I'd reply, but he persisted, reaching for the drawstring of the bag.

"Let me be your flunky," he'd say, urging me with his eyes. "You're the hoopster today, and I'm here to make your life easier."

I'd grin and let him have the bag, which he proudly carried between courts and to and from the parking lot. On these trips he almost behaved like a caddy—silent unless I asked for his input. He knew more about basketball than almost anyone in any gym he ever walked into, but he had no need to demonstrate his knowledge. He knew, innately, that trying to coach me really served only one person: himself. He'd decided that he was there as a dad, not to stroke his ego.

Looking around at those tournaments, I always noticed that my dad was one of the only fathers willing to stand back, play a supporting role. The rest stood in groups, like at a bar, flaunting their basketball acumen as if the point of the tournament was for them to puff out their chests as experts.

"Let me be your flunky" was about remembering that when someone is creating or building a dream, what they need most is your optimism, enthusiasm, and support. What they need least is criticism and self-appointed expertise, which usually serves only to lift you up at the expense of their burgeoning joy and enthusiasm.

"Let me be your flunky" was a dad carrying a gym bag for his daughter, but it was much more. It was a parent supporting a child's dream without centering it on himself.

Chapter 26

KB IS OVER THERE

Turns out, I was the best lip-reader in the family, and the amount of pride I felt about this fact was immodest. In the hospital, in the first days after the tracheostomy, when my dad was trying to say something, I was called over as consultant. If I could instantly decode my dad's sentence, he grinned and nodded, awash with relief and happiness; but if I too was stumped, his face crumbled, as if recognizing anew the chasm separating him from the people he loved. The stakes felt excruciatingly high.

For some reason, my mom couldn't read my dad's lips, and her sadness was palpable. She felt she was failing him. I wished I could transfer some of my lipreading skill to her, like a Venmo payment, but also, selfishly, I wanted to keep it all for myself because it made me feel that my dad and I had a special bond, that we were simpatico again. If someone else was by his bed and he was trying to make himself understood, he almost always started looking around the room for me.

Feeling needed by him brought me so much purpose. I realized that feeling no longer existed for him. He no longer felt needed by any of us. He wasn't Dad, who could troubleshoot our lives; the superhero who once drove from Albany to New York City to install an air conditioner because Ryan was miserable during a summer heat wave. He had been removed from the ecosystem of life, that flow of give-and-take, that delicate balance.

The inability to give was what most eroded his sense of self. And so, throughout the course of his disease, he had cherished the last gift he had to offer: his voice. When we asked him what it was about his days that gave him value, first on his list was consistently "Making you laugh," which he'd always been adept at. But the thing about wit is that by definition, it demands quick and inventive verbal dexterity. It's about whipping the ball *around the horn,* to use a basketball metaphor. Nobody did it better than my dad, and he knew it, too.

Which was why the loss of his voice was too much for him to endure. There was the practical effect of its loss, like something out of a horror movie: He couldn't communicate with nurses if their actions caused him pain. The best he could do was thrash his right foot and hope they noticed. We as a family became his voice, standing by his bed like conductors—*watch out for his right shoulder, it's painful; he can't hold up his neck*—numerous times a day. He would have been willing to endure intense physical pain for years, but he could not abide social isolation, not even for days. Right after the surgery, we could see it in his eyes, a longing to be a part of us again.

I can only imagine how much pain he was in the day after Thanksgiving 2019, when he told us he wanted to die, after he'd been in the hospital, without his voice, for just a week. My wife and I walked into his hospital room to find my mom trying, and failing, to calm him down. On this morning his blood pressure was sky-high and he was sweating. He turned to my mom, then me, and mouthed these four words: *I want to die.*

We kept asking if he was sure, and each time he mouthed back to us *I want to die*. He made sure to form each word carefully, to avoid confusion, even though this sentence seemed to pop from his lips. Slowly, excruciatingly, we would say each word back to him: You. Want. To. Die. After each word, he would blink his right eye (left eye meant no), which was the crude communication system we'd put in place for after the operation.

His hospital bed was angled toward the corner TV because he couldn't turn his head. The chair my mom had slept on was covered in a white sheet. The machine he was attached to had started beeping, signaling his elevated heart rate.

I was relieved, that's the truth. The acceptable thing to write is that I was relieved *for him*, that I was thinking only *of him*, but that would not be true. I was relieved for myself and for my mom and sister, that we had finally reached the end of our time with ALS as the center of our lives.

We worked with the hospital to honor his decision, but arranging to die in a hospital creates miles of red tape, and it wasn't until the weekend that the outline of a plan came into focus. We would transfer him to the ICU sometime on Monday, where we would start the final morphine drip.

The bureaucracy gave us more time together, and on Saturday night just us kids—me, my sister, her husband—were sitting around my dad's bed telling stories. He was helping us, triggering memories with single words that we would decipher from the movement of his lips. Once we were off and running, sharing the memory jogged by his word, he would smile, eyes twinkling.

At some point Kathryn must have slipped into the room and pulled up a chair behind me, at my dad's feet. But our eyes were on him, our hands gripping his. His eyes got big and he mouthed a sentence. We'd had a long run of success, maybe an hour without a desperate miscommunication, and so we were feeling confident. These five words we could decode.

"Say it again, Dad," I said, squinting, focusing. I didn't want to let him down. Often, my brain would translate a ridiculous sentence, related to nothing, and I'd say it aloud anyway just to see him smile.

"Kate likes steak rare," I said, and since this was just Attempt No. 1, he offered the smile I'd hoped for, then mouthed the sentence a third time.

Fuck, I couldn't get it. I looked at Ryan, who shook her head—*no clue*—then back at Mike, who was also baffled. Finally, I noticed Kathryn behind me, and I turned and reached for her; "Hi, my love," I said, turning back to Dad and our twisted game of charades.

He mouthed the sentence a dozen more times, becoming increasingly frustrated, his eyes seeming to drill holes into Kathryn, as if something in her history, or maybe her history with him, would make her more likely to decipher the words. She seemed honored, and was tilting forward to see him better, to prove him right.

All four of us: *Is it something you need us to do? Does it have to do with what we were just talking about? Do you need us to get someone? Are you in pain? Are you trying to say Ryan is your favorite daughter?*

On multiple occasions he made it clear the idea wasn't worth translating, but we were too far along to give up. He rolled his eyes at us: *Give up, give up.* Finally we deployed our system of last resort: one person said aloud the alphabet and he would blink when we reached the correct letter. In this way, we could painstakingly spell out the sentence.

"K…"

"KB…"

"KB i…"

"KB is..."

"KB is o..."

"KB is over..."

"KB is over there."

KB is over there? We all looked at him, looked back at Kathryn (nickname: KB). He pursed his lips and arched his eyebrows: *I told you it wasn't worth the effort.* At first we felt we had followed the treasure map only to find an empty chest, then quickly we started laughing at the ridiculousness of spending that much time—when we had so little left—translating a throwaway observation.

But then my dad did something I'd seen him do a thousand times during his life: he made something simple into something meaningful. Over the next twenty-four hours he incorporated "KB is over there" into his repertoire of sentences and dropped it on us anytime she walked into his room. At first we still had trouble deciphering it, but then someone would say, "Oh, wait—*KB is over there!*" and we'd all look between my dad and Kathryn. Those words became his way of connecting with her, telling her he saw her, that he was glad she was there with him. And since that time I've used the phrase a hundred times. If I'm in a room and someone asks me where my wife is, I smile as I say, "KB is over there." Or whenever we're all together, Mike might say from the living room to the kitchen, "KB is over there."

My dad would have loved to know that even without his voice he created, for his family, another inside joke.

Chapter 27

GEZELLIG

My dad and I got into what would be the most explosive fight of our relationship on the morning of my nana's funeral. A few years out of college, I was finally at an age where I felt empowered, almost required, to go toe-to-toe with him, as opposed to when I was a kid, and mostly just burst into tears. The weakness in our relationship wasn't combustibility; it was the steady erosion of intimacy caused by talking past each other. The fight took place away from my mom and sister, so my dad and I were the solitary witnesses to our undoing. It was our secret.

A miscalculation on my part caused the argument. My dad and I were charged with running an errand, going to CVS to pick up a few extra picture frames so that my mom and her sisters could place additional photos on and around their mom's casket. The night before, I'd realized how contentious a process this actually was: loved ones fighting for space and recognition, each photo and its placement a referendum on how much they loved and were loved, like the seating arrangement at a wedding.

I recognized this behavior as petty, even as I kept score. My error came in assuming that my dad agreed (or even cared) about the ludicrousness of all this, and that we could commiserate on the car ride to CVS. I'd underestimated his stress level, as well as how my comment could be seen by him as causing more pressure during an already difficult time.

"How come my cousin gets *another* framed picture?" I asked glibly, and my dad slammed the steering wheel and threw up his hands.

We sat in the parking lot outside the CVS for a long time, just screaming at each other. In my memory, the van is rocking back and forth, and we're both refusing to back down. He thought I was self-centered; I thought he was a moody asshole. The fight had nothing to do with picture frames.

I always sensed that my dad thought I should care more about family. I was forever missing holidays and birthdays and wakes and get-togethers. "Don't forget today is your grandpa's birthday," he would say, calling me from his car after visiting Grandpa on his way home from work. These gentle reminders could have been just that, although my body would tense up: Why is he telling me this? Does he think I don't call Grandpa enough? Is he also reminding my sister, or does he assume she's more responsible?

My dad lived in the same area in which he grew up; he worked with his brother, Dennis, who had started a financial advising business; he spent winter nights at the basketball games of my younger nieces and nephews. He wouldn't have been wrong to wonder how he'd raised a daughter who couldn't get away fast enough and who made no credible noises about someday returning.

I knew he was right. I should have called Grandpa more. I should have prioritized certain family events. And I knew my annoyance, seemingly directed at him, was really annoyance at being reminded that my priorities were incorrectly ordered. Nothing came before work: I moved anywhere, skipped weddings, missed birthdays. I was unsure about from where, or from whom, my obsession with success came. When I looked around my family, I didn't see it reflected back at me, with the exception perhaps of my mom, who possesses the same ache to leave her mark on the world. *Someday, I'll figure it out,* I told myself. Eventually I would balance my life. But first I needed to stockpile achievements—enough so they could satisfy me for a lifetime. Family would always be there, waiting. That's really how I thought of it: family will always be there, waiting.

So, really, the fight in the CVS parking lot was about imbalance. I'd acted like we were on the same level, both showing up for the funeral, both doing our part, both allowed to bitch and complain. But my dad, I think he saw me as someone who hadn't earned the social capital—within our family—to be talking shit about anyone else, especially not on the day of a wake.

That's how I see it now. At the time, I told myself he was cranky and irritable, and I was the unlucky daughter in his path. We never talked about this fight. And since nobody witnessed it, no one reminded us of it. Inside the filing cabinet of my mind, *The Fight at Nana's Funeral* got tucked away.

On Sunday night, he mouthed a sentence to me. *The fight at Nana's funeral.* He would be transferred to the ICU the next day, at which point we would initiate a morphine drip, and when we were convinced he was deeply sedated, we would turn off his breathing machine. But this was still an unknowable number of hours and a room transfer away, so we could all slip in and out of pretending it might not happen at all.

In high school I ran cross-country, mostly to spend time with my sister, who was one of the best runners in the area. I loved everything about the sport except for the running. I loved the long bus rides to beautiful parks; I loved the tents we pitched like a little village; I loved the assortment of goodies everyone baked; I loved all the smart, quirky people who chose running. Every meet was like a perfect Saturday, except that I knew, at the end of all this joyful communion, that I would be forced to line up in the cold wearing only shorts and a singlet, a gun would go off, and I'd be in pain for 3.1 miles.

Crowded around my dad's bed, surrounded by everyone I loved, I thought repeatedly of that long-ago feeling. The circumstances drastically different, but the energy similar—the volume of it cranked all the way up. I even had a name for the feeling: *gezellig,* a Dutch word not easily translated, but one that captures a feeling of general togetherness, a cozy warmth.

My mom had learned the word her first year out of college, when she and my dad lived in Amsterdam, where he played his first season of professional basketball. They lived in a row house overlooking a canal, and one night, after a particularly lovely party, the wife of one of my dad's teammates used the word and my mom asked what it meant. The woman tried but failed to come up with a precise translation for *gezellig,* thus searing the word into my mom's mind. How incredible, my young mom thought, that more precise language allows you to more precisely experience the world. Language shapes our experience, and not just the other way around. Once I had this word, I realized I couldn't decipher whether it illuminated an already existing feeling or actually created it.

On the last night of my dad's life, my mom, sister, and I stayed overnight in the hospital with him. We rolled in a cot, pushed together chairs, and tried to get some sleep. Every few hours a nurse would enter to give my dad more morphine, but once or twice he stirred anyway and mouthed "I'm anxious," and one of us would go advocate for an extra dose. We were not all needed that night, but we were all in need. We had promised him, when he told us he wanted to die, that we would not let him die in mental or physical agony.

When I would stir awake, I would look around the room and feel deeply in love with all of them. How acutely I missed them, missed us, as we used to be, as I used to see them. Over the years we had been in many rooms together, but we were never *us* again. Ryan wasn't a daughter, she was a mother to her own kids; my dad was a grandpa, I an aunt. Looking around the hospital room on my dad's last night was like looking into a dystopian portal: There we all were, our tight-knit nuclear family, everyone returned to their roles. Except—how had this happened?—we had all aged. The snap of two fingers: twenty-five years. Time isn't linear, it's hopscotch. And I kept jumping back and forth.

I imagined showing this sight to myself in 1995, and how that would have terrified me. And yet here I was, and what I felt was not terror; it was peace. I projected another generation into the future, to myself on my deathbed, and I had this fleeting sense of how I will feel then: *Here I am. Of course. A snap of the fingers.* But we are not meant to hold on to this kind of time travel, and each time I built my own future it instantly evaporated, like fingers through smoke. It felt impossible to keep in my mind, just like the feeling of awe about the universe— *Holy shit, this is all there is*—that blooms and fades in an instant.

So, in those hours around my dad, it was like we created a force field of connectedness, of *gezellig,* of joyful communion, even as we steadily marched toward the starter's gun. Outside the windows of his hospital room a snowstorm was dropping two feet of snow, but inside we burned memories for warmth.

The fight at Nana's funeral. My dad mouthed it again, looking only at me, hoping I could read his lips. My sister and wife and brother-in-law looked baffled, because they didn't know this had ever happened.

"The fight at Nana's funeral?" I said aloud, and he repeatedly blinked his right eye—*Yes, yes, yes.* "Wait, Dad, is that something you've thought about a lot over the years?"

I looked at everyone else and tried to explain. "It was this huge fight we had, outside CVS, about—actually, it doesn't even matter anymore what it was about."

"Why are you bringing that up now?" I asked him.

He looked at me and mouthed, *I'm sorry,* and I said, "I'm sorry, too," and then he nodded slightly and seemed to be processing some form of closure, like the shutting of a file.

I learned, right then, that you'll never know what stays with you, what you'll still be thinking about in the final hours of your life. We can hope that it's all weddings and births and vacations, but what shape will those have without the fights outside CVS? Without disruption and discomfort, the lovely memories become glossy, flattened, like a magazine advertisement—almost like your own life is lying to you. And as much as I dreaded walking to the starting line in my singlet and shorts, I also knew it was that struggle that gave the rest of the day its texture.

I am not Dutch, and it is not my word to define, but now when I think of *gezellig,* I think of an evening filled not just with warmth, but with beautiful melancholy.

Chapter 28

HIGH-WIRE ACT

We are not risk-takers, my family. The idea of skydiving strikes me as absurd, but so too does driving a boat too fast over choppy water, or riding a bike down a mountain trail, or jumping on a trampoline. Even when I'm doing yoga, certain poses feel perilous, pulse-quickening, such as a handstand against the wall. Actually, being upside down anywhere, on a roller coaster or flipping into a pool, makes me nauseated with a sense of vulnerability, the dependability of the horizon spinning away. I've never wanted to live on any sort of edge, and this is a quality I inherited from my dad.

Now that I think about it, nothing in my family was taken to extremes—not drinking, not celebrating, not sadness, not even grieving. My dad liked to say, "Don't let the highs be too high, because then the lows will be too low." This always struck me as rational. The goal, as I saw it, was to exist in a steady state of *pretty good*, even if that meant downplaying exciting milestones—a college scholarship offer, a big new promotion, a wedding anniversary. I started to think of life as a zero-sum game: today's high will be paid for by tomorrow's low, so keeping the feelings of both at arm's length was essential.

I wasn't numbing myself with drugs or booze or sex. No, it was much more oppressive than that. I was dulling future pain by sacrificing present joy. A terrible deal, this one I'd made with myself—and without full awareness of why or when. Picture me, after getting an offer to work at ESPN, barely cracking a smile, saying something deadpan like, "That's such good news, thank you"—never letting excitement blossom in my chest, just so that years later, if I ever got fired, I could tell myself that working at ESPN had never been that important to me, that I hadn't lost that much anyway.

In the beginning, avoiding danger of any kind seemed sensible. But over the years my bravery continued atrophying, and I realized that, like water under a door, fear started creeping into everything. I can remember once standing inside an enclosed gondola and being unable to move away from the center. My mind began unspooling worst-case scenarios, and my heart and lungs felt like they were being smashed together. And that same feeling—heart and lungs in a blender—would happen when I thought of difficult conversations I needed to have with loved ones. Specifically, with my dad.

I've never been a daredevil, and that's fine. But over the past few years I started to worry that my aversion to risk was one symptom of a much broader concern: I'd gradually become less willing to push myself past my comfort zone. Either that, or my comfort zone had become smaller. Once upon a time, when I was younger, I challenged myself, pushed the limits, and turned myself into a professional basketball player. Then, for the next fifteen years, I used that achievement as a mental crutch. I told myself I was capable of testing myself—the evidence, my hard-won college scholarship—but that I was choosing not to anymore, that I was choosing to be kinder and gentler with myself. Voilà: complacency without guilt.

For much of my adult life I've been the person in a fitness class who does only five push-ups when the teacher calls for ten, or who sits out the challenge pose in yoga without even trying. In order for this not to touch my sense of self, I'd constructed a story: that growing up, I physically drove myself every day, so on my list of "character traits," that box had already been checked. I already was that person, even if I no longer behaved like that person. It was like tenure: nothing I did could add to it, and nothing I didn't do could take away from it. Whether I ventured into new territory during a workout was arbitrary, I told myself, and independent of whether I could push myself as a writer, or as a wife, or as a daughter. I was someone who could live in my comfort zone during one endeavor, then shatter it during another.

This story was remarkably sturdy. It took me a decade to realize it was bullshit. I was doing just enough of everything to be *pretty good,* which is a really safe place to live.

For a while, this didn't bother me so much. Our culture's obsession with greatness needn't be my own. But then, one night, I was struck with this scary thought: What if risk-taking, in all its myriad forms, is tied up with empathy? I don't mean risk-taking as in bungee jumping, though for some people that could be the thing; I mean the risky moments we're faced with daily, those small choices when our mind has to convince our body, or vice versa, to go just a little further—the moments when your soul, if you're listening closely, is whispering *You can do this, promise.* Do we work on that sentence a little longer, or is it *pretty good*? Do we handwrite the letter, or is the friendship *pretty strong*? Do we hold the plank all thirty seconds, or are we already *pretty fit*?

Could it be that in these daily moments we're reminded, especially, how hard and beautiful it is to be alive? And if we're aware of how hard and beautiful it is to be alive, then we're conscious that it must feel something like that for everyone else, too.

The first TV show I started doing at ESPN was *Around the Horn* *(ATH)*, which airs five nights a week. It's a sports debate show on which the host—the inimitable Tony Reali—scores the arguments of the panelists, with extra points for pop culture references and well-timed rejoinders. In the fall of 2016, I began doing the show a few times a week, learning the ropes about how it was made. Having watched the show since I was in high school, I was surprised to learn that it was taped. Everything about it had always struck me as spontaneous. But each day, the same process would unfold: a conference call in the morning to go over the topics, articles circulated by the show's staff for research, then an early afternoon "sit-down time" when we would tape the show.

The second time I was on the show was the first time we "busted" out of a segment—that is, the producer stopped the taping, and a few minutes later, we started anew. Sometimes the reason for busting was beyond our control as panelists. For example, the tape of a game highlight was supposed to roll but failed to launch. But at other times, the cause of a bust was a panelist simply forgetting their train of thought or saying something unfit for air. The consequence was minimal, but perceptible: you added, usually, fifteen to thirty minutes to everyone's workday.

About my fifth or sixth time taping *ATH,* I was the cause of busting out of a segment. About midway through my monologue on the New York Yankees, my mind simply went blank. After a few seconds speaking random words while tearing through my brain looking for the thread, I dropped my head in defeat and the producer called out "Bust!" I began apologizing profusely to my colleagues, who assured me it was no big deal, they'd all done the same thing many times.

This specific failure somehow paved a new neural pathway in my body. I can still conjure it: nerves lit up, searing, body radiating from head to toe, teeth set to chattering. It was shame mixed with embarrassment, precisely the sensation one imagines in their night-mare version of public speaking.

A year after I started doing *ATH,* I was asked to fill in as host of *Outside the Lines,* another ESPN show. Pretty quickly, I learned that unlike *ATH, Outside the Lines* aired live. What if what had happened taping *ATH* occurred during *Outside the Lines,* except *on live TV,* with no recourse? I'd become one of those viral blooper videos, like the "Boom Goes the Dynamite" sportscaster guy.

Then a strange thing happened. I did one episode of *Outside the Lines,* then another, then another—and never once did I let my train of thought escape me. There were moments when I could feel the thread slipping away, but the option of stopping the search, of giving up, wasn't even on the table. I knew in my bones that the net to catch me didn't exist. One thought might not directly connect to another, but I would continue speaking until I found solid ground. Pretty soon I realized *the net was the problem.* The net, which should make me feel safe, in-stead gave me permission to give up more easily, to not push through the risky feeling, to not trust that I would find my footing eventually, and to not challenge my mental dexterity and perseverance.

A year later I still needed breathing exercises to calm myself before taping *Around the Horn,* yet while walking to the *Outside the Lines* studio I was focused and present. Alive and confident is how I felt—doing what was, by most measures, the riskier endeavor. I started to believe that during the taped show, I needed to be perfect. When my choice of words, or connecting thought, was slightly flawed, sirens went off in my mind. Then I'd let go and fall into the net. *Well,* I thought, *if it isn't live, then it should at least be perfect.* And when I was on *Outside the Lines,* it was as if my mind understood: we're out here doing something new, risking it all, so let's be kind to us and rise to the challenge.

One pattern dragged me down, the other liberated me. For a

long time this observation applied only to my work at ESPN. It took longer for me to realize its wider implications. My whole life was lived over a net. The net was all around me. I'd put it everywhere. I had the belief that there'd always be another chance—another birthday to celebrate, another chapter of my life to focus on family, another stretch of time to learn a new language, another occasion to talk to my dad, another opportunity to prove I could sit still during life's most heart-wrenching moments.

The net was the voice in my head telling me that now wasn't necessary. Now would be nice, of course, but it wasn't imperative— *Relax, take it easy on yourself, there'll be other chances.* Staying inside my comfort zone, waiting for a sign from the gods, for the stars to align, cost me compassion. Because one effect of believing the net's lie—*Now isn't necessary*—is to pass judgment on those who act; it's the urge to criticize someone taking the bold stroke you're busy convincing yourself to sidestep.

I no longer consider myself risk-averse, even though I still feel queasy looking at a trampoline. I've done the riskiest thing humans can: I've kept my eyes open; I've refused to look away.

In my dad's last months we would sometimes go to the casino along the Mohawk River, a few miles from our house. My mom would drive my dad's wheelchair, and I'd walk in alongside them. To get from the parking garage to the casino floor, we had to take the elevator. The three of us would wait on the patterned carpet, facing the gleaming aluminum doors, then the bell would ding and the doors would part. This was the moment I dreaded: those thirty seconds inside that elevator. All four walls of its interior were mirrored up to waist level; I could escape viewing my own likeness, but my dad could not. As we pushed him inside, I would watch him seeing himself—each time a hollower, sicker version reflected back at him.

I wanted so badly for him to look away. *(Just avoid it, just drop into the safety net, just deal with it later.)* But he never did. He always focused intensely on himself—his eyes a mixture of surprise and sadness. He knew, as I came to know, that closing your eyes is not a solution. It's an avoidance tactic, and a dangerous one, because now that image you evaded lives inside you, unexplored, able to haunt you later. And since your eyes weren't open, your mind can allow the vision to be something it never was.

The night before my dad died, the nursing staff had to transfer him from one bed to another, then move him across the hospital, a relocation we fought against because even subtle movements like rolling him onto his side triggered hours-long breathing crises and immense pain. A team of six, three on each side, prepared him for the move. One of us needed to be present, to translate for him, to articulate which parts of his body must be treated with extra care.

I locked eyes with my dad's and said, "I got you." He blinked his right eye: *Yes.* And for the next ten minutes, ducking under tubes as he was turned, squatting next to him as his machine was lifted, pressing onto my tiptoes as he was wheeled, we looked at each other, fully present, until he was safely inside the room in which he would die.

I didn't close my eyes. I didn't turn away. I saw him clearly—every bit of his pain and fear and sadness. It is the riskiest thing I've ever done, and I've never felt more human.

Chapter 29

THE MANY GOODBYES

And see the bird with a leaf in her mouth
After the flood all the colors came out
—U2, "Beautiful Day"

My dad knew the specifics of how he would die: we would bring him to an ICU room, hook him up to morphine, turn off his breathing machine, and his lungs wouldn't be able to sustain him. Technically, he would die of suffocation, but we promised him he wouldn't feel that part, that he'd simply drift away on a wave of opioids.

The cause of death is birth, as the Buddhist saying goes. We live knowing we'll die. But for most of us this truth only fleetingly bubbles to the surface, then we return to our regularly scheduled programming. We cannot consistently ruminate on our own death and leave enough room to live.

On one hand, as I watched my dad during his final forty-eight hours, I knew his experience was routine. He was dying. But on the other, I recognized his end-of-life experience as exceptional. Not many of us would actually choose, or want, to know the time and date of our death, but he did—even if just a short time in advance.

He simultaneously despised this limbo, while also being desperate for more time in it. For someone who'd always seemed so terrified of death, my dad had certainly been given an extra-large serving.

As we crowded around his bed, I knew better than to ask him to articulate the view from the brink, because I knew what would happen. His brow would furrow, and his eyes would become ominous, like the question itself was drowning him. No release valve existed. Just the buildup of unspeakable—literally, he was unable to speak—emotion.

What he wanted was for us to tell stories, to fill the space with our memories, our voices, our laughter. And to hold his hand. One of us was always holding his hand. I tried to touch him as much as possible, to make up for all the times I hadn't. Months earlier, he had started asking for his hand to be held. Usually it was the middle of the night, which complicated the request. I'd be up and down from the couch, executing monotonous tasks: taking off his breathing mask, putting it on, readjusting it, getting him sips of water, moving his pillows, fixing his blanket, queuing up a new TV show.

Usually around 3 a.m., while I was up rearranging the breathing mask, he would say, "Can you hold my hand for a while?" This meant sitting in the rigid dining room chair next to his bed, but almost always I said, "I would love to hold your hand, Daddy," then we'd sit in deafening silence while I placed my hand on his and rubbed his forearm. He had really nice hands, my dad, with a crooked ring finger from a basketball injury he'd never thought important enough to fix. He'd try to move his hand inside mine, then he'd say, "Can you feel that?" I'd look down at the lifeless imposter that was his beautiful hand and notice a small twitch in the very tip of his right pointer finger. No matter how many times this precise exchange happened, my heart would leap at the slight movement. Was he lifting the finger higher than yesterday? Could the muscle be firing again?

He'd say, "Come on, come on," looking at his hand, concentrating, and I knew he was sending the signal from his brain—*I command you to lift*—and yet the message was lost somewhere inside his body. Where was the signal? How hard was it trying? Could it reroute itself? I thought maybe everything that had turned itself inside out could, just as easily, turn itself right side in. But then I'd remember that wasn't going to happen. The cure would always be just out of reach. It reminded me of childhood, that moment when a balloon gets loose but it's still within range. Somehow you miss it, and so you jump to try again, but then it's floated too high. I don't know if anything is more unsettling than that moment, the balloon drifting up and away, the mind reeling: *Oh, is that how quickly we can be lost? And where will it go now?*

All those nights holding his hand, and only one comes to me clearly. I am sitting in the uncomfortable dining room chair massaging his forearm, and he asks if I can hug him. I tell him I would love to hug him, though hugging him is challenging; I worry about laying too much weight on his chest and crushing his weakened lungs. I arrange myself like I'm playing billiards, one foot on the floor, the other leaning across him, and I rest my head on his shoulder.

He sighs, relieved, like I've lit a fire on a cold night. After a few seconds he starts whispering into my ear: "Katie, my little superstar. You're so good and kind and turned into such a good person. You'll always be my little superstar." The way he spoke, it sounded like a memory, like he was picturing me as a little kid. And I hoped he was. For just those few seconds, I was able to be in two places at once: me now and me then; him now and him then. Our younger selves were wiser; our wiser selves were buoyant.

"Katie," he whispered again.

"Yeah, Daddy?"

"You have to get up now, I can't breathe."

I try not to think of the night he asked me to hold his hand and I said, "I can't, I'm so sorry, I have to go lie down," then collapsed onto the couch. I try so hard not to think of this, just like I try so hard not to think thoughts when I meditate. Yet there they always are. Yet there it always is. During those final forty-eight hours I held his hand as much as I could without being accused of monopolizing the space. Other people loved him, too, I reminded myself. (My mom and sister most of all.)

We loved him so much we were ready to take care of the version of him that couldn't move or talk, just to keep his presence in our lives. But it turned out, very quickly, that he was deciding he couldn't live that way. The day after the tracheostomy, he mouthed, *You were right,* and although I knew what he meant, I pretended I didn't. A few days later, on his eye gaze machine, he sent me a message that read, "You were right about the trach," and I wrote back, "What do you mean?," then added, "More accurate: I don't want to hear what you meant."

A few minutes later he wrote, "OK. Sorry just praising you for your foresight and wisdom at such a young age."

At least a dozen times, I've heard someone thank a musician or author or actor for their work, which helped them "get through a really difficult time." I always scoffed, suspicious that an artist's work could become so vital that it would play a supporting role—not just during a difficult time, but also afterward, in its recollection. How could a stranger become so important during your most vulnerable moments? I thought of it as a transference, an avoidance, the focus taken away from where it needed to be, landing on something safely distant.

It's not as if I was seeking songs and movies as distractions. When your world has been atomized, everything shimmering and unsteady, in this state of disorder you become porous and absorbent—a different you, open in a different way. It's like these atoms have been put in a vacuum and you're floating around, but you sense that if you could just swim to the record player and start the song, gravity would return, the ground would rush to your feet. And so over and over again, you deploy this trick to keep from falling down.

And this is how Kate McKinnon of *Saturday Night Live* became a wall to lean against. During the ten days my dad was in the hospital at the very end, I watched every McKinnon skit, every movie she was in, every late-show appearance. One specific hospital overnight, everyone running on fumes, I stayed with my dad and decided I wouldn't fall asleep. I'd noticed I became increasingly short-tempered each time my dad woke me, but if I could just stay awake, that was less likely to happen. I watched six consecutive hours of Kate McKinnon skits in between bouncing up to help my dad, who was struggling to regulate his temperature and get his blood pressure and heart rate within normal range. This was the last solo overnight I would ever have with my dad, and I never once let fatigue enter my voice, or made him feel guilty about waking me, or told him I was too tired to hold his hand. In the early hours of the morning he found a sliver of calm, and I sat quietly with him, absorbing the peace I could sense he was feeling.

Who cares if it's a one-way street, if it's an illusion? I will always love Kate McKinnon, and she will always remind me of this serene hour with my dad.

The morning he would be transferred to the ICU, we all sat around his bed because we wanted his blessing before starting the morphine drip. We knew he wanted to be told when his last conscious moment would be so he could properly say goodbye, but we foresaw a blurry line, when he'd dip in and out of alertness, making it hard to know when he'd slip under for the final time.

"If that happens, do we have your permission to continue with the morphine drip anyway?" my mom asked. He squinted at us, considering. I thought back to the summer before, when we were at the basketball court and we both realized he'd never again shoot a basketball. It's not always a gift, knowing it's the last time.

Yes, he mouthed.

A parade of family and a small group of friends came through to say goodbye that final weekend. But once we moved to the ICU, it was just the starting five: my mom, me, Kathryn, Ryan, and Mike. And we thought of ourselves that way—in honor of him, because that's how he would have thought of us.

His room number in the ICU was 108, a piece of information that caused my wife to gasp. "That's a sacred number," she told my dad, kneeling by his bed, before we moved him.

At first, as my wife explained the meaning of 108, I thought he'd roll his eyes, but, no, no; he'd revered inexplicable forces such as fate, luck, momentum, destiny. Kathryn was, it turns out, speaking his language.

"So, 108 is an important number in mathematics because the diameter of the sun is 108 times the diameter of the earth, and the average distance between the sun and earth and the moon and earth is 108 times their respective diameters. Some mathematicians believe 108 reminds us of the wholeness of existence, of our place in the cosmic order of things. And in yoga, a *mala* has 108 beads, and the number, we believe, represents spiritual completion."

He smiled, nodded solemnly, like he was honored to be going to Room 108. Unsaid, of course, was that he'd rather not be going at all. About an hour before we moved to the ICU, he asked for his eye gaze machine and typed a short note for my mom to read at his wake. We watched him scan the keyboard with his eyes, slowly, meticulously, selecting each letter:

It was time. I could feel myself weakening. Hands, legs, voice, patience. It was best for me and those around me. Be sad, be angry, but keep doing the things you love. Thank eye gaze for my ability to write this but also its brevity. It was a great run. So many people to thank and so little time and technology. Grab the things you love to do, do them. Sometimes time is shorter than you think. Be sad and swap a flattering story about me.

During that last weekend, he would again mouth, or type with his eyes, the directive he wanted us to follow—the piece of advice he was adamant that we remember. It's now tattooed on my heart: *Keep doing the things you love with the people you love.*

We settled into Room 108, knowing we were still in control of what would happen next. A nurse came by and set up a morphine drip, but my dad was still awake. We didn't know how quickly he would be pulled under, and we weren't ready—he wasn't ready. We didn't start it right away. But he already had a good amount of morphine in his system, so he was drifting in and out. My mom leaned across the top of his bed and cradled his head. She began whispering into his ear, remembering moments that were theirs. Some of them I recognized— I'd heard so many stories—but they weren't my memories, as much as I sometimes felt they were. Yet the story of my parents' lives was smuggled into me, through their DNA, their blood, and as we listened to my mom, I could see the images, shimmering: *Do you remember Corsica... what about that one summer when... how about that night in Amsterdam before... when Ryan was little and... that first Christmas in... at our wedding, after the...* My dad closed his eyes and listened. And whenever we worried that he'd drifted under again, he would smile gently at something she said. He didn't want her to stop. The rest of us swapped seats every so often so we could hold a different hand, touch a leg—get a different perspective.

Eventually the nurse came in and asked if we wanted to start the morphine drip, and we said yes.

We had anticipated the potential blurred line of consciousness, the straddling of here and there. But I had believed, foolishly, that we would know the moment of goodbye as it was happening. I really had thought of it as being like a movie, and just as melodramatic, everything precise and scripted and not at all messy. But we lost control.

We said goodbye a dozen times, each time believing it to be the last, each time watching him drift under only to reemerge, eyes wide, heart rate spiking, as if he definitely didn't want to go yet. It was almost comical, like saying farewell to someone stepping into a revolving door only for them to reappear a few seconds later—again and again.

No matter how many times we said goodbye, nothing changed about our last words. Everything of substance had been said—these words now were the confetti: *I love you; We love you, Daddy; You're the best; It's okay, it's okay; We love you so much; It's okay now; You're safe now.*

I don't remember the last words I spoke to my dad. And I'm glad I don't. Why should one sentence matter more than the millions that came before? Each of us, inside that room with him, had some version of the same final words, and thank god for that.

It tells me there was nothing left to say.

Overtime

FEEL MY MUSCLE (PART II)

Two months after my dad's death, I had a call with a medium recommended by Dana. I brought my phone upstairs with me, shut myself into our home office, and waited until the appointed time. The medium was a woman, a friend of a friend, and she knew little about me: my name, that was it. I was skeptical, not cynical, but more than anything I was excited.

I called at the top of the hour and we chatted for a few minutes. She has dogs, French bulldogs, and they were barking in the background. *That's unusual,* she said, then floated an explanation: *Have you, by chance, ever had a French bulldog?* I had, in fact, and I laughed. *Ah, okay,* she said. *They're saying hello.*

A few minutes passed, and I could tell that her attention was elsewhere, because she started talking to someone else, as if they were in the room with her. *What's that? Yes, mmm, okay, I'll tell her.*

Before she could tell me what was said, I asked, "Wait, is...are you...talking to my dad?" She said she was, though I shouldn't think of it as talking, because the communication is less precise. My dad was doing his best to communicate using energy and images and, when she could pick them up, a word or phrase.

"I understand," I said, even though I didn't.

The things she told me he was saying were spot-on: she heard basketballs bouncing, she asked me if I had written a nice article about my dad before he died (I did). I remained skeptical, though, because I knew a Google search of my name would reveal all these things.

A minute later the woman started laughing at something my dad *(my dad?)* was communicating. I waited patiently even though I felt like I was a beat behind on all the jokes, like I was at the U.N. and I was waiting for my translator to bring me up to speed.

"He's very funny," she said to me eventually. "He just keeps, like, puffing out his muscle and saying, I think he's saying, *'Feel my muscle, feel my muscle.'*

"Does that—does that mean anything to you?"

In college I had a wretched experience with born-again Christianity. The group, and church, I became immersed in seemed driven by judgment and self-loathing rather than love and humility. And when I came out as gay, they made it clear that they would accept me only if I promised to reject my sexuality. *Love the sinner; hate the sin—* that old song and dance.

For the next decade I lost the faith. Not just in the Bible or in Christianity, but in anything and everything toeing the line of spirituality. You lived, you died, and anything that happened between was a coincidence. Still, I wouldn't have called myself an atheist, because that's also an active belief system, and it was dogma in general, not Christianity in particular, that scared me.

Kathryn was the first person to perceive my overcorrection, my pendulum swing from born-again Christianity to nihilism without considering any of the milder options along the way. I had just put my head down and dead-sprinted from one side to the other. Gradually, she pointed out my tendency toward extremes. "Do you think it's healthy, this all or nothing?" she'd say. "Maybe there are gradients worth considering?" She believed in the harmony of the world, the significance of numbers (Room 108!), reincarnation, higher power, empaths and mediums, moon rituals—all of it. And she held these beliefs tenderly, just for herself, not as an outward performance or a way to control others.

Of all these things, my dad believed most in the power of numbers, though he treated that belief more like a superstition, like hopping over the first-base line on the way off the ball field. It was a furtive tip of the cap to the existence of something bigger. In sports, spirituality is often dressed up to look like superstition. Many athletes firmly hold two oppositional ideas: they are both the masters of their fate and at the mercy of the universe. *(The ball just didn't bounce our way...)*

Like many people, my dad noticed and respected the power of one particular set of numbers: 11:11, especially when seen on a clock. He did not specifically believe the number appeared in his life at the behest of a higher power or higher spirit. But he would have said, if pressed, that the number served as a reminder that life is ultimately mysterious, and we should respect the mystery and reach out to the people we love. And that's what he always did. Hundreds of times, I received calls or text messages in which he'd say, "11:11...love u, Katie." (He loved ellipses; they were his favorite punctuation.) When I left for college, to Colorado, which was two hours behind Eastern Standard Time, he started also acknowledging 1:11, saying aloud, "Love you, Katie," and touching the clock, because he knew it was 11:11 where I was.

On the morning of December 4, 2019, he died at 1:11 a.m. I

don't know what that means, if anything at all. My dad, he was as knowable to me as I imagine any dad is to a daughter. And yet, still so mysterious.

Take, for example, the simple fact that a man who was not particularly religious, and had no classical spirituality, restored in me, at his very end, a steadfast belief in a higher power. When I think of my dad now it sparks the same feeling as when I notice the clock reads 11:11: that I'm connected to something bolder and bigger, something that I can't yet imagine.

ACKNOWLEDGMENTS

Just two months after my dad died, I asked my mom if I could write this book. We were at a coffee shop in downtown Charleston and she said, "I was hoping you'd ask me that; I think Dad would be honored." The reasons I'm thankful for my mom are many: for knowing I needed to write this book, for reading through it a dozen times, for writing a beautiful foreword that always makes me cry, for fighting for my dad and keeping him with us as long as possible, for loving adventure and travel and good conversation, for being a wonderful mom and friend and one of the most brilliant people I know.

To my sister, Ryan, and Mike and Henry and Francesca: I love you all. I wish the Big C was here to read *Go, Dog, Go* ("Goodbye!") and call us a half dozen times a day. But we still have one another, and if I'm going to follow his advice and "keep doing the things I love with the people I love," then it'll be with you. Same goes for my best friend, Shawna Hawes, and my b, Kate Scott, and Nevin Caple— whether it's been three days or three months since we've seen each other, knowing you all exist in the world makes it better. To Jane McManus and Tony Reali: The way you showed up for me…I'll never forget it. I love you both.

ALS is a brutal disease, and navigating its tumultuous waters is exhausting. Thank God for places like the St. Peter's ALS Regional Center, and for people like Zach Tonkin and Dr. Roberta Miller (and the rest of the staff in Albany), who are brave and compassionate and honest. Zach: Thank you for answering my calls, even on the weekends, even when I had questions that I knew you couldn't possibly answer. And thank you to Dr. Neil Shneider at Columbia University for his kindhearted attentiveness and genuine warmth. My dad was right when he said you find good people in bad times.

It seems insufficient to call Vanessa Mobley just "my editor at Little, Brown," as she's become a friend and mentor and someone whose perspective and insight on life helps shape me on and off the page. I don't think this book exists without her, as it started mostly as commiseration between two people watching beloved fathers struggling. My dad was diagnosed while we were putting out *What Made Maddy Run* together, so it is not hyperbolic to say Vanessa was there with me every step of the way. Thank you for believing in me and caring deeply about the world and how we can help make it better.

To the rest of the team at Little, Brown—Ira Boudah, Katharine Myers, Ben Allen, Craig Young—it is truly a pleasure to bring books into existence with all of you. Ira, Katharine—your kindness and diligence and passion don't go unnoticed. Anthony Mattero, my agent at CAA, who responds to my (many) texts and emails with assurance and enthusiasm and who saw the potential in this book right from the very beginning: Thank you and let's keep making cool stuff together. To my "other" agent at CAA, Michael Klein: Even though I left the ESPN world, you didn't leave me. Thank you for the loyalty, which I aim to emulate.

Technically, the whole book is a *thank you* to my dad, but it wouldn't feel right to omit him here. Dad: It's such a cliché, but I have a saved voice mail from you that I listen to occasionally, just to hear your voice. You are deeply missed, by me and by many. Our stories were always intertwined, for better and for worse, and now I've just committed them to paper. I hope you approve.

Kathryn Angela Louise Budig, wow...*you* married *me?* I don't know what we expected six years ago, when we first started, but we've certainly received a crash course in life. The good news is that there's no one else I'd rather do it with. I am honored to spend my life with you. Thank you for letting this book breathe, in all the ways I hope it does. If it is real and compassionate and honest, it's not just because you offered me the space to experience those things, but because you cultivated them in me. You, too, hold me steady without holding me still.

ABOUT THE AUTHOR

Kate Fagan is an Emmy-nominated journalist and the #1 *New York Times* bestselling author of *What Made Maddy Run,* as well as the coming-of-age memoir *The Reappearing Act.* She currently works for Meadowlark Media and writes for *Sports Illustrated* and previously spent seven years as a columnist and feature writer for espnW, ESPN.com, and *ESPN: The Magazine.* She was also a regular panelist on ESPN's *Around the Horn* and host of *Outside the Lines.* She lives in Charleston, South Carolina, with her wife, Kathryn Budig, and their two dogs.